The Paradox of Hope

The Paradox of Hope

Journeys through a Clinical Borderland

Cheryl Mattingly

UNIVERSITY OF CALIFORNIA PRESS

Berkeley · *Los Angeles* · *London*

University of California Press, one of the most
distinguished university presses in the United States,
enriches lives around the world by advancing
scholarship in the humanities, social sciences, and
natural sciences. Its activities are supported by the UC
Press Foundation and by philanthropic contributions
from individuals and institutions. For more
information, visit www.ucpress.edu.

University of California Press
Berkeley and Los Angeles, California

University of California Press, Ltd.
London, England

Library of Congress Cataloging-in-Publication Data

Mattingly, Cheryl, date.
  The paradox of hope : journeys through a clinical
borderland / Cheryl Mattingly.
      p. cm.
  Includes bibliographical references and index.
  ISBN 978-0-520-26734-3 (cloth : alk. paper)
  ISBN 978-0-520-26735-0 (pbk. : alk. paper)
    1. African Americans—Medical care—United
States.   2. Chronically ill children—Medical care—
United States.   3. Medical anthropology—United
States.   4. Poor—Medical care—United States.
5. Social Medicine—United States.   6. Medical
personnel and patient—United States.   I. Title.
    [DNLM: 1. Chronic Disease—United States.
2. African Americans—United States.
3. Anthropology, Cultural—United States.
4. Child—United States.   5. Poverty—United
States.   6. Professional-Family Relations—United
States.   7. Stress, Psychological—psychology—United
States.   WS 200 M444p 2010]
    RA448.5.N4M38 2010
    362.198′92008996073—dc22   2010009492

Manufactured in the United States of America

19 18 17 16 15 14 13
10 9 8 7 6 5 4 3 2

To the families who have so graciously allowed us into their lives and to my husband, Steven Heth, who has become my family

Contents

Prologue

In one sense, this is a book about everyone. It concerns the suffering that comes with bodily affliction and the efforts people make to create and—perhaps more important—to reimagine hope even when life has become very grim. As humans, we are all subject to the vulnerability of our bodies. We all suffer. But this book is also more specific, directed primarily to one social scene: the clinical encounter. While clinicians are important here, the main characters are African American parents bringing their children to hospitals and clinics for care. These are mostly very ill children or children with severe disabilities. Thus this is a biomedical story, a race story, and an American story. It is also a relationship story, speaking to the complexities of creating working partnerships between clinicians and families and the trickiness of that effort. I've tried to tell this tale from many points of view: parents, clinicians, and (as much as I could) the children themselves.

This is also a book about ideas, a philosophically oriented anthropology. It offers a proposition for a way to examine hope and, beyond that, social life itself as a narrative practice. In making my case, I move between meditations on big ideas and fine-grained analyses of moments of everyday life. The chapters are filled with stories, but there is significant attention to abstract argument and reliance upon some key philosophical texts. Chapter 2 is especially dense in this regard. This theoretical attentiveness provides a conceptual framework (and its justifications) as a kind of road map before readers enter dense ethnographic scenes filled with small moments and close encounters. These initial schematic arguments allow me to introduce my basic claims and to connect them to scholarly traditions, especially philosophical ones, that may be unfamiliar to readers. For those interested in more detailed discussions of some of these arguments, lengthy notes provide further elaboration.

Finally, this is an ethnography grounded in many years of research. One of the strengths (and luxuries) of philosophy is the careful working through of ideas, but one of its weaknesses (to my anthropological mind) is that philosophers often rely heavily upon very simply drawn examples. Philosophy is not required to do what anthropology does, namely to bring theoretical frameworks into conversation with the complexities of the "real world." So I have also found it important to render close descriptions of social events and situate them within broader historical landscapes, including individual, family, community, and cultural worlds. This close-to-the-ground attention to the everyday offers, as Clifford Geertz famously put it, "the sociological mind with bodied stuff on which to feed" (1973:23). He goes on, in a quote that is still useful to remember: "The important thing about the anthropologist's findings is their complex specificness, their circumstantiality. It is with the kind of material produced by long-term, mainly (though not exclusively) qualitative, highly participative, and almost obsessively fine-comb field study in confined contexts that the mega-concepts with which contemporary social science is afflicted . . . can be given the sort of sensible actuality that makes it possible to think not only realistically and concretely about them, but, what is more important, creatively and imaginatively with them."

Acknowledgments

The cases I present have emerged out of well over a decade of research and the efforts of many people. The kind of study I have done stands at the opposite pole from anthropology's traditional lone researcher toiling in the field by herself (if there ever exactly was such a person). It is born out of the work of many partners over the years, including colleagues, former students, and friends (by no means mutually exclusive categories). First, there is Mary Lawlor: together, we have served as principal and co-principal investigators on a series of grants that have funded this research. She has been a close colleague and friend, a research partner for more than twenty years. She has written a good deal about the complexities of partnerships between clinicians and families in pediatric care. Her formulations and insights into this domain have been critical to my considerations not only of hope but also, more generally, of the immense relationship work that goes into clinical care. Lanita Jacobs-Huey, a linguistic anthropologist, joined our team as a co-investigator in 1999. Her comments, insights, and the nuanced way she speaks and writes about race have helped me immensely in shaping my own thinking.

Then there are the many researchers, graduate students, postdoctoral fellows, and research faculty who have spent some years on the project. Not only have these colleagues been an essential part of ethnographic fieldwork, they have also contributed numerous conceptual insights over the years through our "data interpretation" groups. While no one has been involved for the duration of the project except Mary and myself, many were part of it for three years or more, and some have left and returned to the project, reflecting shifts in our funding and in their own lives. Core ethnographic researchers have been Jeanne Adams, Kim Wilkinson, Kevin Groark, Olga Solomon, Melissa Park, Teresa Kuan, Nancy Bagatelle, Erica Angert, Carolyn Rouse, Alice Kibele, Janine Blanchard, and Courtney Mykytyn. Several other colleagues have been part of the data analysis or have substantially contributed to other forms of research support (literature reviews and the like) that I have benefited from directly. These include Katy Sanders, Juleon Rabbani, Kevin Chang, Amitha Prasad, Anita Kumar, Teresa Kuan, Melissa Park, Jason Throop, Aaron Bonsall, Ignasi Clemente, Cynthia Strathern, and Steven Rousso-Schindler. But there are many others who have worked on this study over the years, graduate and undergraduate students at the University of Southern California who have supported this research in invaluable ways: transcribing interviews and videotapes of clinic and home sessions, videotaping the Collective Narrative Groups, providing technical computer support, or taking care of children while parents talked to the research team. Although I can't name them all here, I want to offer a heartfelt thanks to this dedicated crew.

And then there are the readers, people inside and outside the project who have read various versions of this book manuscript over the years. They have helped me see what I was saying when I myself was often unclear. This is another long list. The most central are friends as well as colleagues: Mary Lawlor, Lone Gron, Melissa Park, Teresa Kuan, and Lotte Meinart. With every one of these friends, there have been "walks and talks" in which I have tried out various ideas to see what would happen to them. Lone and Mary, in their different ways, have been supporters and also incisive critics when my arguments became too confusing and unclear—as they easily do. Mary and Lanita know the families I write about as well as I do. We have spent many hours trying to understand their experiences and their lives, puzzling about them and worrying about them. Uffe Juul Jensen has also played a special role over the years as a friend and sympathetic challenger, asking me essential and critical questions from his own philosophical position.

Finally there are the readers who helped to shape the book in the end. These include Art Frank and Susan Whyte, reviewers whose comments and suggestions were so apt that they actually made the daunting task of revision more bearable. Stan Holwitz also played a crucial role as editor before his retirement, and Malcolm Reed was very helpful in taking over as editor.

None of the chapters in this book, as they now stand, have appeared anywhere else in print. However, versions of some of the cases, and bits and pieces of previously published work, have been integrated within these book chapters. (I should note that often I have changed pseudonyms in various publications to help protect confidentiality of research participants.) Earlier published work where some material from this book has appeared includes: "Stories That Are Ready to Break" (Mattingly 2008b); "Reading Minds and Telling Tales in a Cultural Borderland" (Mattingly 2008a); "Chronic Homework: Social Hopes, Dilemmas and Conflicts in Homework Narratives in Uganda, Denmark and USA" (Gron, Mattingly, and Meinert 2008); "Acted Narratives: From Storytelling to Emergent Dramas" (Mattingly 2007); "Pocahontas Goes to the Clinic: Popular Culture as Lingua Franca in a Cultural Borderland" (Mattingly 2006a); "Reading Medicine: Mind, Body, and Meditation in One Interpretive Community" (Mattingly 2006b); "Performance Narratives in Clinical Practice" (Mattingly 2004); "Becoming Buzz Lightyear and Other Clinical Tales: Indigenizing Disney in a World of Disability" (Mattingly 2003); and "The Fragility of Healing" (Mattingly and Lawlor 2001).

I have presented earlier versions of some of these chapters—or parts of them—in many places and to a range of intellectual and clinical groups, both in the United States and in Europe. Such presentations, and the discussions they engender from the audience, have helped immeasurably in the formulation of arguments. While I could give a long list of conferences, I will confine myself to singling out several communities that, at different times, have played the most significant role—outside the research team, of course—in providing me a space to think things through.

One is a community of Danish researchers, primarily in anthropology and philosophy, at the University of Aarhus. The Center for Health, Humanity and Culture, Department of Philosophy and History of Ideas, under the direction of Uffe Juul Jensen, has offered a crucial intellectual home, even when visits have been sporadic. In the fall of 2009, a joint Guest Professorship in the Department of Philosophy and History of Ideas and the Department of Anthropology and Ethnography at the University of Aarhus provided financial support and an invaluable source of discussions as I revised the book manuscript—especially chapter 2.

A second is the Mind, Medicine and Culture Seminar, where a group of medical, psychological and linguistic anthropologists at the University of California, Los Angeles, regularly meet. I have presented to this seminar on occasion and attended when I could. Several members of this group, graduate students and faculty, have read earlier versions of various manuscripts that have (in some form or another) found their way into chapters in this book. This seminar has been one place that has fostered scholars interested in cultivating person-centered and phenomenological perspectives in their anthropological fieldwork and theorizing.

Though it has been some years since we got together, a third community I want to mention is one that Linda Garro and I organized—we called it the Narrative Group. Anthropology faculty from both the University of Southern California and UCLA with a wide-ranging interest in narrative met about once a month to discuss working papers. Participants were Candy Goodwin, Janet Hoskins, Nancy Lutkehaus, Gelya Frank, Mary Lawlor, and Elinor Ochs. I can still hear the voices of these participants; Elinor originally gave me the idea of considering children's popular culture as a "lingua franca" in clinical care.

I would also like to thank the Bar Ethnography Group (you know who you are) for creating another kind of home, often sorely needed in the midst of writing challenges. My husband, Steven Heth, deserves special mention, not only as a source of support and as a listener to half-formed ideas, but for helping me in all kinds of practical ways, including his inspired idea of using Adam Fuss's work for the book cover.

In addition to acknowledging those who have influenced my thinking through the writing of this book, I want to step back in time to thank some communities and individuals who have played such a vital role in shaping my work on narrative and the phenomenology of illness and healing. I first started thinking about stories as a mode of thought and action in my graduate student years at MIT. As I was beginning to expand my own perception of the narrative, Glenn Bidwell argued with me, encouraged me, and kept giving me more philosophy to read. Donald Schon was very persuasive in challenging the idea of practice as the mere "application" of theories and beliefs. The American Occupational Therapy Foundation, under the direction of Nedra Gillette, launched me into the world of hospitals, chronic illness, and disability. Maureen Fleming became a partner in that research among the occupational therapists.

A Harvard group of medical anthropologists (funded for many years by the National Institute of Mental Health), under the direction of Arthur Kleinman, Mary-Jo DelVecchio Good, and Byron Good, offered me a first entrance into the world of medical anthropology. Those Friday morning seminars—those of us who have taken part in them know what I am talking about—provided a kind of education I had never gotten before. It will be no surprise that I still often reference the works of these scholars as well as many of my colleagues who, at one time or another, also participated in the Harvard NIMH group. Jerome Bruner, teaching at New York University when I came to know him personally, has been both an inspiration and a supporter over the years.

This ethnographic study has been made possible by several major federally funded grants, and I would like to acknowledge them here: (a) "Crossing Cultural Boundaries: An Ethnographic Study," funded from 1997 to 1999 by Maternal and Child Health in the Department of Health and Human Services; (b) "Boundary Crossing: An Ethnographic and Longitudinal Study," funded from 2000 to 2004 (#1 Ro1-HD38878) by National Center for Medical Rehabilitation Research in the National Institute of Child Health and Human Development, National Institutes of Health; and (c) "Boundary Crossings: Re-Situating Cultural Competence," funded from 2005 to 2011 (#2 Ro1-HD38878), again by the National Center for Medical Rehabilitation Research in the National Institute of Child Health and Human Development, National Institutes of Health. The National Institutes of Health also provided supplemental grants that supported two vital members of the research team: Lanita Jacobs-Huey (#3 Ro1 HD38878-02S2) and Ann Neville-Jan (#3 Ro1 HD38878-01A1S1). Additional support has been provided over the years by the Division of Occupational Science and Occupational Therapy under the direction of Dr. Florence Clark.

Finally, I want to thank the many clinicians, children, and family members who have allowed us such access to their lives. There has been such generosity. People have given time, a willingness to speak frankly, often about very difficult matters, and—in the case of families—invitations to all manner of family events. I have never carried out research where people invited me in to this extent. It would not have been possible for me to write this kind of book, to tackle the questions I do, without such openness. Although, to protect confidentiality I cannot name them personally, I hope that my gratitude can be heard.

CHAPTER I

The Lobby

The first time I interviewed Andrena was in the main lobby of a large urban hospital. A cavernous space. Strangely dark, even formidable. Later I could see that the gloom had its comforts. A good place for quiet crying, or for staring into nothing. High ceilings, clusters of permanently fixed plastic chairs lined up in rows of three or four, or set together in L shapes. Chairs as neutral as could be, in tones of beige and practical brown, placed neatly on the wall-to-wall gray carpet. Some leafy potted plants (plastic too, but the realistic kind) helped divide the room into smaller waiting areas. The lobby always felt empty, odd for a hospital full of children. At one end, almost unnoticeable, was the receptionist's desk—not the busy center of this clinical space, as one might expect, but far away, giving the impression of a waiting room with nothing to wait for. Of course, I could have some of these details wrong. This interview took place many years ago, the fall of 1997, and the hospital was redecorated two years later.

I didn't mean to talk to Andrena in such an anonymous place, but where could I go? This was new research in a new city. Sometimes you can find a cozy enough corner even in a big hospital, but I didn't know my way around. And Andrena's very ill daughter was lying in a room three floors up, so Andrena was not about to go far. I had met her only once, a week earlier in her daughter's room on the east wing. I was introduced by the friendly speech therapist who thought Andrena might be willing to participate in the study my colleagues and I were doing.

When I saw Andrena that first time, she was sitting on a chair, holding the hand of her daughter, a little girl of four and a half whose shaved head was barely visible above the white sheets of the bed. The small half room was jammed with people. People standing, sharing chairs, leaning against the radiator or a wall. The child's father, a grandmother, an older sister, an uncle, a cousin. Before we entered, the speech therapist told me that the parents were separated and Andrena was the one to ask. After some quick introductions, I directed my attention to her. To my surprise (her daughter looked so frail and her mother held her hand so tightly), Andrena smiled and agreed immediately to participate. "Sure, sign me up," she said. "I'd be glad to help." I left a few minutes later with the plan for our first interview.

So there we sat, Andrena and I, in the twilight of that lobby, diagonally faced in our plastic chairs, my tape recorder perched between us. There is one thing I have noticed about interviewing people in the crisis of life. Many of them don't need much in the way of pleasantries. Time has changed its speed; it has become concentrated, portentous. It may be too fast or too slow, but it is never luxurious. Better, then, to get straight to the point. Andrena was one of those, I could see, who wasn't in the mood for leisurely opening remarks. "So," I said, "can you tell me the story of your daughter's illness up until now? Just begin at the beginning, wherever that might be for you?" And then she started to talk.

She talked for an hour and a half, with very few questions from me, and there were no wasted words. One episode of that first long story offers me a beginning too. The more I have considered it over the years, the more it has haunted me, or perhaps beckoned me. After nearly a year of struggling to find out what was wrong with her child, who was growing increasingly ill, Andrena finally got a diagnosis. The relief at being taken seriously by clinicians was quickly replaced by the terror of what she found out. Her daughter had cancer, a brain tumor. As if that news weren't terrible enough, she was pulled aside by one physician who announced that the particular type of cancer her daughter had was "the worst kind." Here is how Andrena put it:

> This one doctor, a lady doctor, she came to get me to explain what they were gonna do . . . And she came and she took my daughter and myself to this one room. And she really—Lord, she had me going crazy because she told me, she said, "Oh, I'm so sorry." I said, "So sorry? Did you hear something else?" And she said, "Well, you know that's the worst one that a kid could have. It's the highest-risk kind." And I said, "Oh my God!" I started

saying, "Oh, no. I'm dreaming. I'm dreaming. I'm dreaming." I just kept saying, "I'm dreaming," 'cause I was picturing it was, like, it's not real. This is, like, something on TV or something . . .

Her nightmare offers a central image for this book.

Andrena's nightmare seeped through the whole of her life, and, as she gradually discovered, there was nothing to do but learn how to navigate in it, even learn to make it a new kind of home, a home where she struggled to hope. Hope offered another sort of dream, an intimation of possibility for a better life even in these grim circumstances.

This book is a meditation on hope grounded in a thirteen-year ethnographic study of African American families—parents like Andrena— caring for children who have severe and chronic health problems or disabilities, as well as the clinicians who serve those children. Hope, that "waking dream" as Aristotle called it, concerns imagined futures (Miyazaki 2004; Crapanzano 2004). Its direction is toward what may come to pass. It cannot be predicted—it is a future of "what if." Paradoxically, hope is on intimate terms with despair. It asks for more than life promises. It is poised for disappointment. Here is how the French sociologist Henri Desroche concludes his consideration of hope. Citing Roger Bastide, he offers this definition: "just a simple pause on a long path that stretches towards who knows what horizon, that retreats with every step we make toward it, towards its promise of light and clarity" (1979:171). With even darker irony, Desroche continues: "Hope as it is drawn by Kafka: 'The Messiah will come only when he is no longer needed. He will only come one day after his advent. He will not come on the day of the last judgment, but on the day after'" (1979:177).

Hope as an existential problem takes cultural and structural root as it is shaped by the poverty, racism, and bodily suffering endemic to so many of the families I write about here. For the people in this study, especially the parents, hope emerges as a paradoxical temporal practice and a strenuous moral project. Biomedicine offers no cure. For many children, the prognosis is bleak. Thus cultivating a hopeful stance is paradoxical; it involves an ongoing conversation with embittered despair. To hope is to be reminded of what is not and what might never be. Family members speak of the call to hope as a moral call, bound up in views of what it means to live a good life, to be a good person. Many have spoken repeatedly about the need to hope, and especially about working to have the "strength" to hope, even when times are hard. I have heard countless conversations where family members and friends encourage one another to keep up their hope. Why is hope so important? Why is it required? What kind of vision of reality does it offer? I could quickly see that it was not the same picture clinicians often cautioned against; it has rarely seemed to me something as simple as delusion or denial. For these families, hope has represented a stance toward reality that requires careful cultivation.

While clinicians and their voices appear throughout this book, my primary focus is on the parents (fathers at times, but especially mothers and grandmothers), who care for these children and work to negotiate health care with clinical institutions. The families I focus on are those I know the best personally, people whom I have seen in many contexts over the years and whom I have come to care so deeply about that my relationship with them has changed how I see the world.

Andrena's news about her daughter's cancer brought with it not only fear but, as we shall see, an imperative to hope in the face of that fear, and in the face of an unknown future that stretched in front of her. I will consider dreaming that comes when you might least expect it, the terrifying nightmares that serious illness or tragedy can precipitate. Even more, I will consider what may be done with such nightmares, the work to make them habitable, to find within their terrifying terrain quieter moments, even small lush pleasures. Andrena and her daughter settled on the couch, watching Disney's *Pocahontas* for the twentieth time, illness temporarily at bay. A trip to the beach on a hot afternoon while her child splashes in the waves with her cousins, a four-year-old like any other. A quiet joke shared with the oncologist when the latest MRI looks better than expected. Her daughter waking unexpectedly from a coma as Andrena prays that God will give her more time to say goodbye. These dramas, large and small, constitute the narrative shape of hope, hope that is not merely cherished or passively received but actively cultivated, practiced.

Perhaps it is the sheer level of suffering that has made this practice of hope stand out in such a marked way. Even in cases where a child's diagnosis is not life threatening or especially physically dangerous, the sheer chronicity of the situation has brought its own dangers. There are no simple solutions. Living with any significant disability, especially when it is coupled with poverty and racial stigma, can be grim work. From one view of reality (a "realistic" perspective), it is, in fact, cause for despair. And despair is precisely what families fight against. They see despair not as realistic but rather as having its own kind of delusion: a comforting delusion that nothing more is required, that the future is fated and they can simply "give up." (They sometimes worriedly attribute this perspective to the clinicians who treat their children.)

How is it that the families and clinicians I speak about here confront this paradox of hope? I am especially interested in the families on this matter, for they, more than the clinicians, struggle with it: How to cultivate a practice of hope that is bearable, despite its elusive promises, its retreating horizons, those darkest times when the suffering is so excruciating that any advent, any salvation, is already too late? How to find a way to hope that will be supported by clinicians and in clinical settings where expensive or even adequate care may be denied—both realities of contemporary health care for many Americans?

HOPE AS A PARADOXICAL BORDER PRACTICE

When it comes to serious illness and disability, hope is a familiar topic. Many anthropological and sociological studies have emphasized the disruption and despair—the lack of hope or struggle for hope—that can accompany chronic and serious medical conditions.[1] Scholars have explored the cultural shape of hope in a variety of contexts, examining the way patient, family, or clinician views of hope "articulate . . . with a society's cultural interpretation of hope" (M. Good et al. 1990:60).[2] Having to adopt an optimistic or hopeful attitude even when the prognosis is grim, as is sometimes culturally required, can put tremendous burdens on patients or family caregivers. Cultural contexts also shape patient-clinician communication about hope—often a fraught topic. Clinicians, too, struggle with how to maintain their own hope and how to convey and "regulate" the hope of their patients: How to give patients a "just right hope"? How to deal with a patient's "denial"? How to help patients find new things to hope for in their future even without the possibility of any medical cure?[3]

The rise of new biotechnologies has provoked new reconsiderations of social hope and clinical care. On the one hand, emergent technologies have helped to fuel health disparities between rich and poor on a global scale, a phenomenon described by some scholars in classically dystopic language. Technology emerges here as a kind of Frankensteinian monster (Lock 1997:238). But the development of innovative biotechnologies has also produced a much more optimistic discourse of hope among other scholars, a hope that has linked forms of democratic and political processes to science and technology itself (Haraway 1997; Rose 2007).

My own starting point for a consideration of hope is grounded in the lives of particular persons and intimate moments of family and clinical life. I consider hope as located not primarily within biotechnical practices or dominant discourses that engender optimism or tragic pessimism (depending upon one's view) but rather, first and foremost, in highly situated practices of people struggling to live with chronic medical conditions. Hope most centrally involves the practice of creating, or trying to create, lives worth living even in the midst of suffering, even with no happy ending in sight. It also involves the struggle to forge new communities of care that span clinical and familial worlds. This is why I have chosen to speak of hope as a *practice,* rather than simply an emotion or a cultural attitude.

I will consider the practice of hope not only as a personal struggle of parents like Andrena but also as a critical aspect of the health care encounter. Poverty and race figure largely into it. I explore how a group of African American families, many of them poor, traverse clinical spaces when their children have serious, chronic, and sometimes critical medical conditions. These navigations through the fog caused by all-consuming suffering are made more menacing by the uncertainties and dangers facing marginalized minorities who seek care in the health systems of the United States. I also consider these navigations from the perspective of clinicians who at times find themselves confused and uncertain about how to provide care or how to connect with families far removed from their own class and cultural background. Hoping is no mere personal affair when it comes to health care in a multicultural urban hospital. It is a border activity. Thus the central question for this book is: How is hope cultivated in a border zone? How does this border practice shape hope for parents, children, and clinicians?

It has become quite popular to talk about life on the borders. Borderlands are perhaps *the* central figure of the contemporary social imaginary. Across a whole range of disciplines, the recognition that social worlds are porous, that boundaries are fluid and contested, and that objects and people are bound together or travel in all manner of unexpected ways continues to inspire our imagination and provoke our attention. In some cases, this has meant a literal focus upon a particular geographic spot, cartographically defined, where one can pay special attention to sites of heightened commerce among actors who are culturally diverse—large, multicultural urban areas, for instance, or the spaces around national boundary lines, zones of war, refugee camps, travels of the displaced across tenuous political boundaries, and the like.

But borderlands need not be so visible on any map. They may also designate spaces defined by *practices* that bind people together who otherwise wouldn't belong together. It is in this practice-based sense that I am using the term *borderland*. It designates that flexible space in which healing is carried out, not only by health professionals, but also by patients and families. The narrative acts I will speak about help to shape this borderland and reveal the fluidity of this space and its connections to geographical and institutional sites that are far removed from any clinic: homes, churches, even Chuck E. Cheese and Disneyland.

In this book, I focus on the task of creating borderland communities and how deeply the practice of hope is bound up with this struggle. I approach this problem through a particular theoretical lens that I call *narrative phenomenology*. Briefly, I have three overall aims. One is an analysis of hope as a clinical border practice, based upon this long-term ethnographic study that has focused upon the multiple perceptions surrounding illness, disability, and healing held by family members, clinicians, and the children they care for. A second objective is to offer a narrative phenomenology of practice that not only recognizes the macro structural dimensions of our social existence (the way discursive regimes are embodied and played out in everyday social practice) but also foregrounds the personal, intimate, singular, and eventful qualities of social life.[4] A third, related ambition is to demonstrate an ethnographic methodology—narrative phenomenology as a kind of research method—that is deeply intertwined with the narrative framework I present.

This is a mixed-genre work, a philosophical anthropology that has its abstract theoretical moments but is also filled with stories. It is primarily through the stories that philosophical—perhaps I should call them existential—questions are raised, questions about the human condition and the place of suffering and hope in it. I will focus upon small moments of everyday life, paying close attention to a gesture, a phrase, an argument, a joke—the pervasive, largely invisible stuff of ordinary social interaction. And in doing so, I will try to paint portraits that are reflective of the personal and social histories in which people live. In that sense, this is a book about the intersection of race, chronic illness, and clinical care in the United States. Yet I do not intend this work as some kind of definitive race story, or a book that speaks only or uniquely about the experiences of African Americans. While the cases I present are sometimes marked by features that make them singular to the

African American experience and to the construction of race or disability within clinical encounters, my intention is to open an existential window onto the relationship between suffering and hope, exploring hope as a practice at once personal and communal. I mean to offer "concrete universals": that is, particular people and events that paradoxically, in their very concreteness, imaginatively reveal something about the struggles of many people, including ourselves.

THE LOBBY AS CULTURAL, HISTORICAL, AND IMAGINATIVE SPACE

I opened my book in a lobby, a space I find especially fitting because I am going to tell travel stories, stories about struggling to create homes where no one lives, to make families (or at least travel companions) out of strangers. I will be writing about "dwelling-in-travel" (Clifford 1997:2), a space of "friction"—of "contingent encounters" and "interconnection across difference" (Tsing 2005:4). When James Clifford meditates on travel as a " 'chronotope' of culture" (1997:25), he gives us an image: the hotel. Hotel "as station, airport terminal, hospital: a place you pass through, where the encounters are fleeting, arbitrary" (1997:17). However Victorian the overtones (conjuring up, as Clifford remarks, gentlemen travelers from an earlier era), it is a useful image. I have it a bit in mind when I consider the lobby. Not a bourgeois chandelier sort of lobby but just the kind you find in bus stations, airports, and, of course, hospitals. If urban hospitals quintessentially exemplify culture as a border zone (as I shall argue presently), then their lobbies offer a front-seat view of culture as a boundary space, a place intended to be temporary. Leaving there, after all, is the primary point.

When you are in a lobby, chances are you are waiting. And not comfortably either, in the lobby I have in mind. Poor and even middle-class families who have very sick children spend quite a lot of time in such lobbies. There is a great deal of waiting to be done when caring for the sick, or in being sick yourself. Lobbies are supremely liminal spaces. You aren't even visiting yet. You are only waiting for a visit. Lobbies, even when well guarded, don't exactly belong to anyone (a notable no-man's-land). In a hospital, they are familiar frontiers. Everyone passes through them from time to time, unlike its many secret spaces where only a few are allowed to enter. Frontiers, by and large, precipitate "encounters between strangers of whom none come to the meeting with the permission to set the agenda in their pockets" (Z. Bauman 1999: xlix). I would not go so far as to claim that all of cultural life can be summed up by this trope. "Motility" and "non-rootedness" may not exactly be the "'primary reality' of culture," as some suggest (Z. Bauman 1999: xlv). But they very pointedly mark the cultural scene I investigate here.

In exploring hope as a border practice, I rely upon a conceptual reframing of culture that has special salience for my purposes, one that has emerged over the past few decades as part of the refiguration of culture, a shift from anthropology's traditional task of elucidating "the crystalline patterns of a whole culture" to a focus on "the blurred zones in between" (Rosaldo 1989:209). The lobby provides such an apt trope because culture has come to be imagined as a site of travel. It is the name of a land one passes through as much as lives in, characterized more by hybridity and liminality than by any uncomplicated citizenship. As a scene of travel, it is attended by experiences of estrangement and displacement.[5] Out of this has come a new kind of social common sense, one that abandons "old ideas of territorially fixed communities and stable, localized cultures" in favor of "apprehend[ing] an interconnected world in which people, objects, and ideas are rapidly shifting and refuse to stay in place" (Gupta and Ferguson 1997a:4). In this resituating, culture emerges more vividly as a space of encounter than of enclosure. Or, put somewhat differently, enclosure itself is increasingly treated as one element of encountering and—very often—conquering spatial practices.[6] But borderlands are not totalizing; rather, they are "spaces of contradiction and disorder, as well as sites of cultural fluidity, identity making, and diverse and marginal forms of citizenship" (B. Good et al. 2008:22). Border crossing is a necessary, if treacherous, business in such fluid spaces.[7]

The lobby, with its in-between, transient character, is metaphorically apt in a second sense. The travel stories I tell concern encounters that have their temporal place within ever larger narrative horizons: they are *historical moments*. They belong as episodes not only within personal, familial, and institutional lives but within national and global ones as well. These travel stories are moments within a colonizing history that spans (even conservatively) three continents and three hundred years. Two historical horizons have particular salience to my topic. One is the rise of modern Western medicine itself, a story that has been told and retold and made especially famous as a dystopic narrative in Foucault's work.

A second history, covering a roughly similar time period, concerns the colonization of the Americas and the importation of African slaves to work on newly founded plantations. The construction of the black body is, of course, an integral part of America's cultural history. Race, and quite specifically racial designations that divide black from nonblack, are "written into daily lives and experience in America" (Goldberg 1997:10), essential to the making of the modern American subject. As we know, these histories have intersected in an especially pernicious way for African Americans. Out of the development of a slave society in North America emerged an accompanying "scientific" medical perspective that became a tool for defining the black body as, essentially, biologically Other compared to the white one. Medicine and the emerging biological sciences helped to imaginatively construct the black body as particularly frail and needy.

This vaster historical race story is vividly present in my metaphorical lobby because so many hospital encounters I describe are encounters across racial divides where participants see themselves or find themselves designated as both culturally and *racially* Other. The history of slavery, race, poverty, and illness lives as a menacing shadow for the families I write about. While I will describe many clinical encounters that reveal its centrality, the history itself will appear only as a shadow. Not all stories can be told at once or with equal clarity. Thus this vaster history is only intimated, gestured to, as I cast my eye on more intimate and immediate scenes. But though it is not explicitly detailed, it is palpably present. It can, for example, be heard in the voices of parents who still cannot shed this legacy of racism or escape the play of race in clinical care.

This practical problem that families and clinicians face speaks to another key feature of culture reconceptualized: the *interpolation of cultural difference and culture making* as mutually constitutive events. "Culture," Lila Abu-Lughod writes, "is the essential tool for making other" (1991:143). The production of cultural difference becomes acutely visible in border zones, creating charged and antagonistic spaces. They are where cultural politics play themselves out, in a particularly heightened way, where the cultural is represented as *difference*. Culture emerges as a "contested category and . . . site of ideological and political struggle" (Mahon 2000:469–70).[8] As many have argued, cultural identity is produced only in the moment of cultural differentiation.[9] Postcolonial, feminist, and race theorists have led the way in much of this theorizing of the borderland. Cultures, Homi Bhabha declares, "recognize themselves through their projections of 'otherness'" (1994:12). The creation of difference is a largely negative capacity, a pernicious cultural virus that turns others into Others.[10]

Travels in Clinical Border Zones

The urban hospital, as I have already suggested, is a quintessential cultural border zone. Because of its cosmopolitan nature, the practice of hope in clinical contexts is very much connected to the problem of understanding one's fellow actors, one's interlocutors. It is not difficult to see that such a border space will be rife with misunderstanding. In border zones, actors find themselves uncertain about what others are up to and struggle to be understood by their interlocutors. While much of life may be fraught with ongoing misunderstandings, interpretive trouble is particularly pernicious in clinical spaces where a great deal is at stake.

Much of the work in medical anthropology has explored transactions within biomedical encounters marked by cultural confusions and misunderstandings—border talk, in fact. Even where there are no differences of race, ethnicity, language, nationality, social class, gender, or other obvious social markers, the gulf between those who inhabit what Paul Stoller (2004) calls the "village of the sick" and their professional healers is, in itself, enormous. We can see this with poignant clarity in physicians' tales of their own illness experiences, and how far these take them from the safety and familiarity of hospital life experienced from the "other side," the land of the well. And of course it is especially and ominously present in the encounters I describe in this book, where families and patients do, indeed, come from social worlds that are distant from those of many of the key health professionals who treat them.

If the practice of culture is so bound up with a practice of Othering, of identifying cultural difference in a thousand subtle and unconscious ways, this is of special importance in health care. In clinical encounters that cross race and class lines, worries over being misread constitute major threats. Misunderstandings are magnified to intense proportions in situations characterized by both cultural difference and high stakes. Cultural identities constructed by race, class, gender, and other potentially stigmatizing markers take on profound meaning here. After all, hospitals are places where things are very much at stake for many of the social actors. What might be a small slight or a confusing conversation in another context can take on enormous importance under these heightened circumstances. To feel slighted by one's doctor when one is seriously ill is not the same as being slighted by the grocery clerk.

Traveling in such a clinical border zone means confronting cultural difference. In the world of clinical encounters, the patients or families are most obviously travelers in the "exotic" land of the hospital, where they encounter unfamiliar languages, rituals, and expectations about how to act their part. But these travelers also confront the problem that *they* may appear unfamiliar or exotic to health professionals. Worse still, they may appear as "familiar strangers," prejudged and slotted in categories where they are dismissed, invisible, neither known nor deemed worth knowing. Parents may emerge as "won't step up to the plate" fathers or "not too educated" mothers, characterizations that challenge everyone's ability to create partnerships necessary for effective care.

Perceptions of difference can precipitate a number of charged scenarios. At its polar extreme they can lead to what Michael Taussig speaks of as the "horror story of hospitalization" in which "the clinical situation becomes a combat zone of disputes over power and over definitions of illness and degrees of incapacity" (1980:9). By contrast, border encounters in hospitals can lead to imaginative borrowing, syncretic inventiveness, the creation of common ground; they may have their creative and even generous moments (A. Frank 2004). These dramatic possibilities are made more complex precisely because this is travel in border territory. This means that it is not always clear just *whose* territory it is. When is one the traveler and when is one on home ground? How can groups who mark themselves as different come to share a territory that is commonly traversed? It may be true that clinical spaces "belong" to the health professionals much more than to patients and families, but things get more confusing when it comes to the patient's body. The body itself emerges as "border territory" in the health care encounter. Sometimes this sense of body as borderland is a central part of the illness experience (Hahn 1985:87–98).

Cultural travelers like Andrena suddenly find themselves faced with trying to understand and navigate the foreign world of pediatric oncological care. She has new languages to learn (languages of disease, of insurance forms, of rehabilitation goals, of X-rays), new social spaces to traverse (radiology labs, oncology reception desks, physical therapy mats), new roles (the patient's mother, the home co-therapist), and new technical competencies to master (how to administer chemotherapy shots to her daughter at home, how to do the occupational therapy home program, how to become deferential to novice clinicians even when she has acquired better mastery over some of these technical skills than they possess).

Most complex, she has the task of trying to create effective partnerships with a vast array of health care providers, from oncologists to lab technicians to hospital receptionists. She must cross race and class lines to do so. This is a task fraught with interpretive challenges. Yet it is one Andrena often effectively confronts. Her successes illustrate the hermeneutic proposition that misunderstanding is not the end point of dialogue but its necessary beginning. While there are countless instances in this book of misunderstandings that only deepen as parents and clinicians attempt to communicate and negotiate with one another, there are other moments that reveal this dialogical possibility of movement toward understanding and the creation of common ground.

The efforts of many of the parents and clinicians point to how they can offer spaces for *cultural imagination and reinvention*. Cultural difference and cultural production may go hand in hand, but in these marginal and contested spaces, to follow Bhabha's provocations, culture reveals itself in its fluidity as well. For it is at the "significatory boundaries of cultures, where meanings and values are (mis)read or signs are misappropriated," as Bhabha (1994:34) writes, "that culture offers itself up for thought." And "friction" sometimes turns out to be the mother of invention (Tsing 2005). "The clash of power and meaning and identities is the stuff of change and transformation" (Ortner 1999:8).

While calling upon contemporary postcolonial and race therapists to consider border zones, I also return to an older theoretical conversation within phenomenological hermeneutics to investigate how Othering occurs in clinical encounters and how it leads to the creation of dramatic experiences that may instigate cultural reinvention. In doing so, I foreground the dialogical nature of encounters (and experience as a kind of "dialogue with Otherness," to paraphrase Hans Georg Gadamer [1975]), in order to investigate such everyday matters as the preunderstandings that actors bring to encounters and the dangers and failures of experience in charged moments that only serve to harden prejudgments and prevent any creation or recognition of mutuality. I find this philosophical approach especially fruitful in investigating the politics of hope in clinical border zones because *experience* is accorded a privileged place in the analysis. As someone who wants to speak of border spaces not only as shared by discursive formations but as produced through the intimacy of personal and intersubjective experiences, this theoretical framing serves me very well.

Blues Hope as a Border Practice: Political and Imaginative Landscapes

The border zone as a space of Othering has been especially consequential for African Americans. In 1970, Ralph Ellison offered this insightful analysis:

> Since the beginning of the nation, white Americans have suffered from a deep inner uncertainty as to who they really are. One of the ways that has been used to simplify the answer has been to seize upon the presence of black Americans and use them as a marker, a symbol of limits, a metaphor for the "outsider." . . . But this is tricky magic. Despite his racial difference and social status, something indisputably American about Negroes not only raised doubts about the white man's value system but aroused the troubling suspicion that whatever else the true American is, he is also somehow black. (quoted in West 1993:3)

The idea, intellectually pervasive within contemporary social theory, that race is a matter of cultural (and politically defined) convention is rendered especially powerful by African American writers who have talked about how they have come to see themselves as "black" or "negro" or "colored" or "nigger" only through the eyes of others, white others in particular. "I remember the very day that I became colored," writes Zora Neale Hurston in a 1928 essay entitled "How It Feels to Be Colored Me" (quoted in B. Johnson 1985:319).

The powerful African American experience of being Othered has not only brought a history of racial shame and political and economic oppression. It has also provided another legacy: an "anticipatory imagination" that is tied both to struggle and to community building. One could call it, following Cornell West's (2008) description, "blues hope." Here, we can see that my metaphorical lobby offers something else, figuratively speaking. It intimates an imaginative space marked by temporal uncertainty. One waits in a lobby not only for a person, a place, an activity, or some news, but for the future itself. Temporally, lobbies are spaces of anticipation, of the not-yet. In this sense, they suggest another kind of border zone, what Vincent Crapanzano refers to as an imaginative frontier. Such frontiers "extend from the insistent reality of the here and now into that optative space or time—the space-time—

of the imaginary. It is this realm that gives us an edge, at times wrenching and painful, at times relieving and pleasurable, on the here and now in all its viscous immediacy" (2004:14). As Crapanzano notes, while scholars have been very engaged in considering political and global borders, they have been neglectful of imaginative horizons, and especially of what he calls "anticipatory imagination" (2004:19).

This is especially unfortunate for the study of suffering, which demands—or ought to demand—attention to imagination. Hope lives in an uncertain place, in a kind of temporal lobby. It points us toward a future we can only imagine. This imaginative and uncertain space of hope becomes acutely visible in the African American experience.

In a book published a few months before Barack Obama's election, West put it this way: "America finds itself looking to its blues people again to provide vision to a nation with the blues. That is a source of hope. Yet hope is no guarantee. Real hope is grounded in a particularly messy struggle and it can be betrayed by naïve projections of a better future that ignore the necessity of doing the real work. So what we are talking about is hope on a tightrope" (6). An African American vision of hope that is not easy commitment to a "blind optimism" but an arduous struggle against fearsome obstacles has become part of a national story, though one often hidden from public sight. This "blues" vision of hope that West speaks of has recently been given a particularly public face because of the election of President Obama. The rhetoric he used and that came to surround his campaign, while specific to a particular event in American history, is remarkably useful in shedding light on something enduring in America—its complex love affair with hope itself.

Hope, as many commentators have noted, has historically been a dominant theme in American life. In its simplest and most naive expression, Americans have long been associated with a national insistence on taking an optimistic stance toward the future. Every American is familiar with an American Dream that promotes an "against all odds" mentality and insists upon a "you can be anything you want to be" cheeriness. This cultural stance has been blamed (with good reason) for rampant individualism and a blind unwillingness to accept structural inequalities produced along class, race, gender, and ethnic lines. This secular political and economic dream is also heavily marked by America's religious legacy, particularly its Christian heritage, in which hope has figured as a key virtue, one of the three (along with faith and love) that constitute the bedrock of espoused Christian values.

A "can-do" ambition, the insistence on "not sinking in the world" that de Tocqueville had already identified in the nineteenth century as America's primary cultural directive, might seem to express America's only vision of hope.[11] Yet a more subtle ethical and relational picture of hope is also part of the American tradition, one that has particular roots in the African American experience and its Christian traditions. Obama's rhetoric provides a vivid illustration. In his watershed 2004 keynote address to the Democratic National Convention, Obama distinguished hope that is merely "blind optimism" and "willful ignorance" in the face of social problems like unemployment and health care from a hope that is "more substantial." He begins his elaboration of this "more substantial" hope with the African American experience, which he then seamlessly links to the struggles of other Americans: "It's the hope of slaves sitting around a fire singing freedom songs; the hope of immigrants setting out for distant shores; the hope of a millworker's son who dares to defy the odds; the hope of a skinny kid with a funny name who believes that America has a place for him, too." He goes on, to thunderous applause: "Hope in the face of difficulty, hope in the face of uncertainty, the audacity of hope: In the end, that is God's greatest gift to us, the bedrock of this nation, a belief in things not seen, a belief that there are better days ahead" (Obama 2004).[12]

While Obama does not relinquish a promise of progress, he also introduces the tougher language of uncertainty, of struggle marked by risks and difficulties, one where hard work will be required and sacrifices will need to be made. He draws upon a rhetoric that is familiar to many Americans, in which hope is a challenging practice, one that does not come at the price of blindness to the real difficulties life poses. This is not a hope rooted in scientific progress, economic expansion, military might, or more shopping but one version of a very American homespun populism continually identified with the struggles of the poorest segments of society and a civic responsibility to work for a common good. This political vision, especially as voiced by many African American leaders, is also deeply associated with Christianity. This is not surprising, given that the church has offered African Americans the single most powerful institutional base for its political battles for civil rights and freedoms.

A "blues hope" is not merely otherworldly, however, despite its spiritual roots. Far from it. It speaks especially to the practice of hope as community building, as border crossing. When Obama borrowed a phrase from Reverend Jeremiah Wright, the "audacity of hope," he also used it to speak specifically to the American possibility of creating community across America's borders and conflict-ridden polarizations. What is audacious about this hope? The belief, against all odds, in the possibility of creating community out of conflict. "That was the best of the American spirit, I thought—having the audacity to believe despite all the evidence to the contrary that we could restore a sense of community to a nation torn by conflict" (Obama 2006:356). Obama has insisted time and again that hope has to do with finding threads of commonality that bind us together and creating a political practice that serves those ethically defined goods (Atwater 2007). He proclaims: "Alongside our famous individualism, there's another ingredient in the American saga, a belief that we are all connected as one people. . . . It is that fundamental American belief, it is that fundamental belief—I am my brother's keeper, I am my sister's keeper—that makes this country work. It's what allows us to pursue our individual dreams, yet still come together as a single American family" (Obama 2004). These proclamations link hope in the most profound way to a civic and ethically construed responsibility to reach across divides, contributing to recent discussions of hope across a variety of disciplines in which "hope has emerged as a way to redefine the ethical contours of the social and the relational" (Miyazaki 2008:5).

The backdrop of America's racial story between blacks and whites, and our enduring struggles as a nation to come to grips with this divide, is deeply implicated in the Obama message of hope. This racial story so infused the Obama presidential campaign that, as journalists frequently pointed out, it hardly needed to be made explicit: "I, you, we can make history, he says, by turning the nation's sorrowful racial narrative into something radiant and hopeful" (M. Powell 2008:1).[13] Obama's speeches are yet another reincarnation of earlier American, and specifically African American, voices of leaders and writers who have confronted America's racial and economic divides and have tried to build political activism on the hope of healing the country's racial wounds by recognizing a fellow humanity and struggling for a common good. Here, for example, is Richard Wright, writing in 1941: "The differences between black folk and white folk are not blood or color, and the ties that bind us are deeper than those that separate us. The common road of hope which we all traveled has brought us into a stronger kinship than any words, laws, or legal claims" (quoted in West 1993:17).

RETHINKING HOPE: A PERSONAL STORY

For the past thirteen years, as I have gotten to know parents, children, and clinicians in urban hospitals, I have seen ways that this same vision has implicitly infused clinical encounters. And I have seen, too, how often it fails to materialize, how often it is thwarted, how fleeting it can be. Hope, as it has emerged on a grand political scale, shaped by voices as powerful as an Obama or a Martin Luther King, is also present—if one only looks closely enough—in the eloquent words and deeds of parents like Andrena. A good deal of this book concerns the immense and complex work that parents, and sometimes children, do to create healing dramas in the midst of disability and serious illness in their own lives and to bring these into the clinic. Those border travelers struggle to instill and cultivate hope in everyday clinical encounters and in partnerships with clinicians, generating complex practices of "border crossing."

The considerations of hope in this book mark something of a personal journey. I started thinking about hope in a clinical setting in the mid-1980s when I began to study the practice of occupational therapists. I became gripped by the problem of what healing might mean for those with chronic conditions (which rehabilitation professionals like occupational therapists specialize in) when curing is a rare possibility. In my study of these clinicians, I gradually came to realize that another and perhaps more basic way of considering this was to see it as a problem of hope. What was worth hoping for when one was suddenly confined to a wheelchair after a car accident or had lost one's speech as a result of a stroke? These questions haunted clinical encounters, though they were rarely voiced out loud by either clinician or patient.

In this early research, I concentrated primarily on the efforts of the occupational therapists to involve their patients in rehabilitation activities that somehow engendered hope, that spoke (generally tacitly) to future possibilities of a life that could still be cherished. This was not the clinicians' language, I should hasten to add. To speak in such terms would have sounded rather lofty, even religious or existential, hardly the voice of the clinical chart. But occupational therapists often talked, sometimes schemingly, about the skill needed for "motivating patients." And they worried about patients whose hopes were "unrealistic" as well as about those who seemed to have "given up" hope altogether.

In the books I published based on this early research, *Clinical Reasoning* (Mattingly and Fleming 1994) and *Healing Dramas and Clinical Plots* (Mattingly 1998a), I considered how therapists worked to create "healing dramas" in the midst of clinical sessions. I defined a healing drama as the configuring of therapeutic time into acted narratives. These acted stories projected possibilities for future lives and selves. One of the most subtle aspects of clinical dramas was their temporal complexity. What happened in the moment of therapy as some kind of enriched present did not matter as much as what that moment portended for a future lived quite outside the world of the clinic. Sometimes the mundane activities of a therapy session, however trivial they might seem in and of themselves (taking a ride in the new wheelchair down to the nurses' station, turning pages of a magazine with a mouth-stick when one could no longer use one's hands, trying out a favorite pasta dish in the rehabilitation kitchen), were transformed from mere tasks to portentous dramatic moments. They suggested that there might be some way to create a worthy life even with a body diminished by disability. In short, they offered moments of hope.

This research prompted me to revisit the hermeneutic phenomenologists I had read as a graduate student and their exploration of significant experience (e.g., Gadamer 1975; Heidegger 1962; Dilthey 1989; Ricouer 1984, 1985, 1988). I could see from my observations of therapists' work and from their informal discussions of "best practice" that for some of them the creation of significant experience was a vital aspect of effective practice itself. It was part of the "art" of therapy, a kind of "underground practice" (Mattingly and Fleming 1994) that could not be reimbursed or documented in the clinical chart despite its centrality to the efficacy of clinical care. In describing this unauthorized aspect of practice, therapists would speak of their concern that "something happen" in therapy so patients would experience sessions as personally meaningful and motivating. For the occupational therapists, this was a practical problem, often expressed in their desire to transform their patients from passive recipients of care to active participants in their own recovery.

On the basis of this study, I made the claim that significant experience was not merely passively received in dramatic form, as can sometimes be suggested by the philosophical phenomenologists, but that actors themselves (like some occupational therapists and patients) may be concerned to create significant experiences for themselves and others. They may try to make certain kinds of stories come true, to create certain kinds of dramas, while avoiding others. This concern that something happen—that time become "eventful"—may be directly linked to the efficacy of clinical practices, providing a culturally shared motivation to create dramatic meaning in specific kinds of encounters.

It was also evident that while therapists might wish for a certain kind of experience to unfold, they were not able to control events or the responses of their patients in order to enforce a pregiven script. In fact, it was commonplace wisdom among experienced clinicians that only novices thought such a thing possible. Good therapists, it was generally agreed, had to know how to "read the situation" and how to "change gears," discerning, in the moment, how patients were responding to the session. Excellent therapists knew how and when to make shifts, even when to abandon treatment plans altogether, if things were not going as anticipated. Experienced pediatric therapists have been especially adamant about the need to develop this sort of improvisational capability in working with children. You have to "capture their attention," they will say, or there is no chance that therapy will work at all.

Although I spent most of my time trying to understand this from the perspective of the therapist, it also became increasingly clear how important the patient's responses and instigations were in shifting clinical time into these more eventful and dramatic moments. And in the interviews I did with patients early in my clinical research, especially with some of the young men with spinal cord injuries whom I got to know, they too spoke of their rehabilitation sessions not so much in the language of acquiring adaptive skills as in a language that was all about their own personal struggles to accept life with devastatingly altered bodies. For them, much more than for the clinicians, learning discrete skills paled in the face of their experience of living in these new bodies. To the extent that rehabilitation therapy mattered to them at all, it was primarily because of the experiences created in therapy time. There were the terrible ones—the time when a trip to the bathroom in the new wheelchair showed them just how much of their bodies they had lost. And there were the fragile hopeful experiences—the time when putting on a shirt by themselves gave them a sense of possibility that went well beyond the specifics of any particular skill.

By the end of this research among occupational therapists, I could see how much their practice involved the work of hope in clinical care. I could also see that if I wanted to understand this work of hope more thoroughly, I needed to carry out a different kind of research study.

There were many questions I could not answer from inside the clinical world. If small clinical moments sometimes portended hope, what happened to these hopes when patients left the hospital? Did they and their family caregivers struggle to find hope at home? In what ways? Did the little hopeful moments of therapy time intersect with the work of hope in home and community contexts? How did hope change over time? What could these home contexts tell me about the clinical moments I had called healing dramas? More basic still, what *was* hope as acted in such transformative dramas? Was it an optimism about a happy ending? A narrative of progress? Already my work among chronically ill patients suggested that hope was more nuanced, less linear, perhaps even something darker. Certainly I could see that for patients it encompassed much more than, and fell well outside of, the confines of a clinical hope that rested on what biomedicine could offer.

To think about all this I needed a different research design, one that focused more on patients and families and less on clinicians and their perspectives. I also wanted to consider hope, healing, and suffering in broader political and social contexts, raising crucial issues of power, class, race, and economics that I had not foregrounded in my earlier writing. For all these reasons I worked with colleagues, especially Mary Lawlor, to develop a much broader set of research projects designed to "travel" with patients and family caregivers between clinic, school, and home. We also chose to concentrate on minority populations plagued by greater health disparities and significantly worse health outcomes than those faced by middle-income white Americans, thus foregrounding issues of race, power, and often social class. My consideration of hope not only as a part of clinical care but as a border activity emerged from this series of research studies that moved across the social spaces of clinics, schools, and homes.

In this research in Chicago and Los Angeles, I found myself plunged into the world of the urban poor, learning to find my way around unfamiliar African American neighborhoods in a city even more intensely racially and ethnically divided than Boston, where I had once lived and taught in underclass urban classrooms for violent teenagers. In 1990, I received a large federal Department of Education grant to carry out an ethnographic study of African American and Mexican American children with learning disabilities to explore disparities and "cultural issues" in education for minority children with special needs. I had assembled a small team of researchers: anthropologists, education specialists, and occupational therapists. Along with other researchers on the team, I spent my time in special education classrooms in several Southside Chicago schools. For the first time, I got to know parents as I went to the homes of the children we followed, trying to find out what it was like for them to raise children with disabilities. I was stunned by the centrality of cultivating hope for those living within oppressive social environments. From the parents, I gradually came to absorb a complexity of perspective that I had not had before. Out of my earlier experiences as a (largely ineffective) teacher of children in great difficulty, I had been left with a kind of helpless despair about the possibility of change for those at the bottom of the social ladder. I had somehow assumed (and it sounds so ridiculous to say it now) that because I couldn't change anything, there was no change to be had.

When I later returned to poor urban neighborhoods and interviewed special education teachers in Chicago, they often seemed to share a similar pessimism about the children they taught. But the parents, many of them, offered a different vantage point. Life was difficult. There was no doubt about that. But there were possibilities too. I spent quite a lot of time at the kitchen table talking to one mother whose son was tagged "severely learning disabled" and who would likely now be diagnosed with autism. (In the early nineties, children in poor black communities—especially boys—were seldom given a diagnosis of autism. Instead, they were likely to be handed either diagnoses of general retardation and developmental delay or ones that categorized them as emotionally and behaviorally disturbed.) His mother rejected these school labels, describing him as "slow" and also "special." For her, his specialness had nothing to do with being in special education. Instead, it had to do with a certain gift to commune with the spiritual world. "He can hear things the rest of us can't," she would tell me, looking fondly at her son playing in the next room. Once when I came to do an interview, her son had a cousin visiting and they were playing together. "Oh," his mother said, "that's Shareen, his 'adopted twin.'"

"That's what we do in my family," she explained at my puzzlement:

Slowness tends to run to some members of my family, you know. Has for generations. So, we pair up the slow person with someone else in the family, a cousin, a sister or brother, something like that, and they become a kind of twin. They help the one who is slow, like my boy. You could say it's their family job.

She gave an example:

I have an aunt who is slow too. She was only a couple years older than me and she couldn't pass her grade when she was in high school. So then she was in my grade. Well, my folks made sure we were in the same classroom together. When she failed some of her courses, I set out to fail mine as well so that I could go to summer school with her. That's so she wouldn't be lonely or have kids tease her too much. I could look out for her.

She also mentioned a nephew of hers who lived around the corner. His parents were sending him to Arizona with a cousin, another slow child, his "twin." He would leave his family and live with his cousin's family, who were moving there from Chicago, so that he could stay with this twin.

This mother told these stories matter-of-factly. It was just what one did, just ordinary life. Such creative strategies for protection and care, not to mention self-sacrifice, opened a whole new world of possibility to me. Things could seem hopeless from the perspective of a professional—a teacher, a school psychologist—but families could be crafting homemade "therapies" to try to take care of their own. Another mother I also got to know had a child she described as "having a lot of emotional problems." (He was also in a "severely learning disabled" classroom.) "The thing about him," she said, "is that because he's not quick, he's not so likely to get in a gang. They aren't going to want him because he's not fast enough. So that's one good thing." She sighed. "But, then, if he's not in any gang, who is going to protect him on the street when I'm not there? He won't have others to look out for him, so he's just a target." She went on, explaining how she tried to solve this problem:

> Okay, I had an idea. He needs to know some basic things to be able to look out for himself because, you know, I'm not as well as I once was. I have diabetes. I'm not always going to be here. So, I set up a little store here in the house where he can sell candy and soda to the neighborhood kids. He learns to count change, to take care of money, and the kids get to know him. He learns some street skills. But he's here, where I can watch over him, not out there on the street where kids will steal his money.

Hearing such stories—and watching parents at home with their children—I not only confronted my own blindness as a teacher and community activist but began to see how social science can be equally blind. Things can also seem hopeless from a theoretical perspective if one isn't careful—if one faces the deleterious combination of disability, racism, and poverty in America and sees only the overwhelming, apparently overdetermining social structures that seem to ensure the reproduction of dramatic inequalities. It would be foolhardy, especially in this particular historical period, to ignore the devastating machinery, both global and national, that perpetuates chilling economic and political inequities. But it is equally foolhardy to neglect the ways even those who are most oppressed locate and cultivate "resources of hope" (Williams 1989) that offer reasons to live and to act.

Through research in Chicago and especially in Los Angeles, I have had not only to rethink hope as a category but also to modify my understanding of what a "healing drama" looks like and why it can matter so much to patients and families. If, in my study of occupational therapists, it sometimes seemed to me that I was importing a foreign language in my glosses of clinical work (especially my talk of healing dramas, transformative journeys, and anticipative narratives), I changed my mind when my focus shifted. As I spent more and more time trying to understand chronic illness and disability from the perspective of patients and especially of their families, there was plenty of talk about hope, and about healing as a personal, familial, and sometimes even communal journey. There is perhaps nothing surprising in this, given the pervasiveness of discourses of hope as related to illness and healing in American popular culture. Such discourses gain particular weight and salience when connected to American Christianity and in light of the role of the black church for African Americans as a religious, cultural, and political institution. It is significant that the African American families I speak of here are nearly all Christian. Most belong to fundamentalist faiths. But this fact can be deceiving. The subtle ways hope is practiced and cultivated among these families cannot be reduced to a mere instantiation of dominant American discourses, including those associated with evangelical Christian traditions.

The realization of my own blindness to these powerful and subtle practices of hope has propelled me to develop research strategies and theoretical frameworks that can uncover them, practices that are likely to be hidden or misinterpreted by clinicians and scholars alike. As I have turned my attention increasingly to patients and families over the last decade, I have realized that in emphasizing the creation of significant experience from a clinical perspective, I was describing and seeing only the tip of the iceberg.

RESEARCH IN A CLINICAL BORDERLAND

The primary study that informs this book began in January 1997 in Los Angeles and ended (officially anyway) in June 2009. It was initiated with a federal grant that Mary Lawlor and I wrote based on research we had done in Chicago. From our own individual and shared studies, we had long recognized how central it was for families and clinicians to create partnerships in providing pediatric care to children with chronic medical conditions. In addition to confronting a host of political and economic problems posed by an unwieldy and unwelcoming health care system, clinicians and parents often felt personally challenged to find good ways to collaborate, especially when they came from very different social backgrounds. There were many sources of trouble. Mary and I wanted to understand not only where and when difficulties arose but also when things worked well or challenges were surmounted. We proposed a study that would focus upon African American families whose children were receiving care in major urban clinical sites that served ethnically and racially diverse populations.

We began the research in Los Angeles by contacting occupational therapists in a few clinical settings, from small outpatient clinics to major urban hospitals. Both of us were known in the occupational therapy community, and we counted on being able to build upon this. Through our contacts, therapists in several of these sites put us in touch with African American families whose children they were treating. During the first few months of 1997, we gradually settled upon three primary sites and recruited an initial thirty families into the study. While at first this recruitment depended upon occupational therapists, as soon as we were settled into these clinical spaces we met families in many other ways. Waiting rooms proved an especially useful spot, since waiting is often such a long business. Children themselves would sometimes come over to see what we were up to as we sat in waiting room chairs taking notes and trying to get our own bearings in these unfamiliar settings. When we approached families, some were eager to participate, some signed on with trepidation, and others refused. Over the years we have followed over forty families, though trying to keep the total number at any one time to about thirty. Some families whom we got to know during the early months of the study have been part of the research for its entirety—more than half have participated for at least a decade. A few have been part of the project for only two or three years. While the federal funding has ended, to speak of this research in the past tense is a misnomer of sorts, for it is not really finished. We promised families that we would continue to have a yearly "family reunion" where we could all meet and catch up with what had been going on in our lives. In April 2010 we held our first reunion.

Many families came, some traveling from as far away as Las Vegas (where they had relocated) to participate.

Mary and I have by no means been alone in carrying out this research. Right from the start we hired other researchers with backgrounds in anthropology or occupational therapy who have played a primary role in recruiting families, collecting data, and discussing how to interpret the data. Thus this has been a team project. Members of the team have changed through the years with the exception of Mary and myself. We have been at its helm, or tried to be, for its entirety. In the acknowledgments I have named the many researchers who have been part of this team, a list of names that is itself a paragraph long. While there are considerable challenges in managing a major research project and trying to do ethnography "at home" with a large, multidisciplinary team, one primary reward is the multiple perspectives introduced by various members of the group. Another is that a great deal more data can be gathered than could possibly be undertaken by any single researcher. But a third is perhaps most important. As team members, we have been able to support one another over the years in trying to live with, or live beside, families and children who have at times undergone immense suffering. I, for one, would simply have lacked the courage or fortitude to carry out this kind of research by myself, even on a much smaller scale.

The People in the Study

We began by recruiting clinicians from the multiple sites where we were doing research, and they then introduced us to families. But very quickly, as we became involved with families, things shifted and we recruited clinicians that families introduced us to, ones who were treating their children. In this way, dozens of clinicians have also become part of this study. When families have moved from clinical site to clinical site, we have tried (where we could get permission) to include these new sites in our study; thus this is very much a multisited study. It also includes a broad array of health professionals: surgeons, oncologists, radiologists, lab technicians, pediatricians, social workers, nurses, nutritionists, physical therapists, speech therapists, health care aides, home health nurses, special educational teachers, psychologists. Demographically, they have predominantly been Euro-American and middle class, though there is certainly some diversity, including Asian Americans of various ethnic backgrounds, Mexican Americans, and a few African Americans.

In recruiting families, our criteria for "qualifying" were quite broad. Initially we focused upon early childhood, so we admitted only families who had children between birth and eight years old at the time of recruitment. We were not, however, disease focused. We rejected such biomedical typologizing in favor of a category that was more phenomenological and more practice oriented—having to do with chronicity itself and the border work that this gives families and children. Thus the children in our study cannot be grouped into a particular disease or disability category. Rather, they have shared certain commonalities of "illness experience" because of suffering from a serious, chronic illness or disability. Children and their parents have also shared (or did share at the time of recruitment) a similarity of practice in several senses. Care has meant frequent visits to an array of health care professionals. Furthermore, families and children have been faced with "chronic homework"—the need to provide care or to carry out health programs at home. Another commonality is race. The fact that the families are African American has meant that there has been a shared racial designation and that for many, seeking care for their children has involved negotiating racial boundaries and racial designations.

Despite these very broadly defined commonalities, differences in social class, in family culture, in level and type of clinical condition, and in personal lives has meant that there has also been a great deal of diversity among families. Attending to this diversity as well as to commonalities has been an important theme in our research.

A few words about why Mary and I chose to follow African American families. From a social justice perspective, African Americans stand out in a very significant way. While the problem of creating partnerships between clinicians and patients (or family caregivers) is by no means exclusive to minority groups, the racial history of the United States means that when interpersonal difficulties arise the specter of race is always present. And this is not merely a phantom. For decades, dramatic health disparities between African Americans and whites across a whole range of diseases have been documented; in most cases this gap is consistently wider than for any other minority group.

These disparities have been linked to two overarching factors. One is the political economy of health care, that is, the persistence of poverty for a large sector of the black population and the structural connection between race, social class, and quality of care. A second concerns what are often called "communication barriers" between health care professionals and African American patients. The most basic problem here is trust. Creating trust between clinician and patient is a significant factor in the effectiveness of health care, especially for those with chronic conditions. A host of research studies have documented the persistence of mistrust in relationships between health care providers and African American patients. The structural and the communicative are intertwined. Poverty plays an enormous role. For those on public aid or without their own physician, emergency rooms are more often used for routine health problems. This means that patients are receiving care from clinicians who do not know them and in clinical situations where clinicians are likely to be harried and exhausted. Emergency room waits are infamous; patients and families are also likely to be frustrated by the time they actually get to see someone. Not, all in all, a promising circumstance for trust building.

Some researchers have speculated that it would be easier to create trusting relationships if clinicians and patients came from the same racial demographic. (And there is some strong evidence for this.) But even if African American patients might more easily trust, and be trusted by, African American clinicians, structural factors enter here too. Urban health care facilities in which a larger portion of clinicians are also African American are routinely underfunded and often poorly staffed because they are generally located in underclass neighborhoods. These communities do not receive the same level of financial assistance from city, state, or private resources that is given to their comparatively wealthier counterparts. And if they are located in poor neighborhoods with higher levels of violence and sicker patients, they are much busier and more overcrowded, with exceedingly long waits in the emergency room.

Where African American patients have a choice, they may opt to get care at hospitals with better resources, even though there may be few African Americans on staff.[14] This became very evident in our study, where many families sought care for their children in hospitals with state-of-the-art technology, less crowding, cleaner halls and rooms, and stronger reputations for having well-trained staff. But this meant that the clinicians treating their children (especially physicians and rehabilitation therapists) were far less likely to be African American. Thus the challenges of crossing boundaries and creating partnerships across race and, often, class divides have been especially heightened for African

American patients. (I have more to say about this in the chapters to come, especially chapter 3.)

Narrative Phenomenology as Research Method: Ethnography of Events, Personal Lives, and Clinical Institutions

In some ways this study shares features typical of an ethnographic tradition, including getting to know a small number of people well, participating in their lives, situating ourselves in a few locales where we could observe the comings and goings of people, and using multiple methods of data collection. But other, less familiar features of this design have turned out to be instrumental in providing a grounded basis for developing a narrative phenomenology of practice. Looking back, it has become clear that the way we carried out this research has been extremely influential in the conceptual framework I have developed, one that moves analytically from the micro to the macro, from the personal and interpersonal to the institutional. Why is this so?

Person-Centered Ethnography

First, although we wanted to have something to say about health disparities as these pertained to African Americans, we were committed to carrying out ethnography that did not attend solely (or even primarily) to how social categories and subjects were produced. We began, instead, with an approach that was much more "person centered." We tried to do what Douglas Hollan has so nicely articulated, to recognize the "importance of grounding our discussions of human experience in the compelling concerns of our subjects' everyday lives. Because the flow of experience is contested, indeterminate, and emergent, we must follow our subjects through time and space, and across different cultural domains, and in so doing, discover what is at stake for them in the course of their daily lives" (2001:55).

From the start, we were determined to attend to how families and children experienced living with disability and illness, learning to navigate the health care system, struggling with their own suffering, and creating lives they deemed worth living. What kinds of matters were most at stake for them? How did these change over time? And what about the clinicians? What were their struggles? How did they define a good clinician, a good patient, what healing might mean? In the context of these personal, familial, and often highly specific and variable struggles and concerns (which we could not know beforehand), we then wondered about social categories: How was expertise produced? What about race, class, or gender? What kinds of categories emerged, were resisted? In what ways and under what circumstances? These were important questions, but these were not our first questions. We did not presume that they were primary to the parents and children whose experiences we were trying to understand. In fact, I write about hope in this book because this, rather than race or class, has seemed to me the central concern from their perspective.

This is ethnography over the long haul, and the impact of this longitudinal design cannot be overestimated. It has allowed us to follow children and families as they change over time. Temporality itself has emerged in a significant way. I have been able to explore concretely and in the context of people's lives certain philosophical claims concerning the phenomenology of human time and the place of narrative in shaping it. Our long-term engagement has revealed a great deal about clinical encounters as events in family lives, about the multiple perspectives that families and clinicians bring to these encounters, and about how healing itself comes to be reimagined and redefined through the course of an illness or a child's life. It brings home the social nature of illness and healing, how much illness (and disability) is also a family affair. As the anthropologist Myra Bluebond-Langner notes in her ethnography of families caring for children with cystic fibrosis, family life is intimately related to "pivotal experiences or events" in the ill child's own illness trajectory (1996:13). Even the possibility of recovery is a family matter.

Event-Centered Ethnography

We have focused great attention on social action and on the interactions between clinicians and families, adopting common techniques of "microethnography," especially videotaping family events and clinical encounters where possible. This has allowed us to return to these scenes again and again and do fine-grained analysis of a few minutes of interaction. Home events include birthday parties, funerals, graduations, and other pivotal temporal moments as well as everyday activities in family life. I have always relied upon videotaping as a key element in my research because it allows such close attention to the details of social action. In this project, we have continued to refine ways of recording and interpreting video data throughout the years. We have sometimes borrowed (loosely) from the tools of linguistic anthropology to help us refine our ways of attending to the small details of social interaction. This book includes dozens of snippets of these videotaped moments, which reveal the centrality of this microethnographic focus.

In adopting an event-centered approach, we were concerned to understand events (especially clinical events) from multiple perspectives. Rather than focusing on the perspective of one of the types of actors in clinical interactions (say patients, family caregivers, or clinicians), we wanted to understand the interactions as the product of multiple points of view. We tried to get at this not only by paying close attention to the interactions themselves but through our interviewing. As much as possible, we did what we came to call "event-centered interviewing": that is, separately asking clinicians, parents, and sometimes children to "tell us what happened" in a clinical encounter that we had also observed or filmed. Events enter in another way. We tried to discover the sorts of activities that mattered most to families and children, accompanying them to such things as drill team practice or soccer matches if these were important family events.

We also spent a good deal of time asking parents (and children, as they got older) to tell us stories about crucial events in their lives. We worked to explore a child's illness or disability as one subplot in personal and family lives and, for this reason, carried out repeated life history interviews. This attention to the personal has been instrumental in helping me see how deeply people locate themselves in ethical projects of Becoming (to borrow from Martin Heidegger) that are very much related to the practice of hope. I have witnessed parents, in particular, come to understand their lives and fates and hopes differently as their lives (and the illnesses of their children) have changed.

Interviewing has been especially suited to the exploration of storytelling as a mode of reflection upon past events. We have heard some stories again and again, stories that change in tenor and tone as they are relived in new present moments. We have also heard "anticipated stories"— stories that speak to what participants imagine will come to pass (my child's first day of school, when my child will be out of the wheelchair, etc.)—and have been able to witness some of those "future times" as children have gotten older. We have then been able to hear stories that participants tell about moments that have become part of history rather than expectation. This storytelling, even when it is focused upon events, reveals a great deal about personal and shared family lives.

This long-term research has offered us a much deeper understanding of why certain moments in the clinical encounter matter so much to parents and children and what kinds of exchanges turn out to be important to these partnering efforts. It has enabled us to connect minute intense moments of "significant experience" to what might appear (especially to clinicians) as routine clinical moments, ones that never show up in the medical chart but speak to the lives of children and families well beyond that encounter.

One unique feature of our research design that has provided a window upon particular events and on biographical lives is the invention of the Collective Narrative Group. When we began this research, Mary and I thought it might be a good idea to see if some of the families wanted to participate in an advisory group. We organized two different family groups, with the idea that we might be able to do a kind of collective interviewing of people who decided to attend and that they might also have some advice or reflections upon the themes that were emerging from individual interviews and clinical and home observations. While not all of the families who signed up to be in the study came to these groups, those who did became very attached to them.

We began these groups a few months into the project and continued to meet three or four times a year. Our poststudy yearly reunion simply continues this tradition. To be frank, at the beginning I thought this was a good idea mainly because federal funders might take to the idea of having a family advisory group. (Federal grant funders often seem to like hearing that you are going to be getting some advice.) But to my immense surprise, these groups have been the source of some of the most powerful data we have collected. They have come to be borderland communities in their own right as families and those of us on the research team have made our own temporary family-like community. So much has happened in them that I could probably devote an entire book simply to exploring how they have evolved since we began them in 1997 and how family members have come to use them for their own purposes. But here I will confine myself to giving a cursory description of what they entail.

Mary and I have co-led them, a tricky facilitation in which we have tried to ensure that everyone who speaks feels listened to and respected even when the things they are saying make others uncomfortable, angry, or annoyed (a feat we have not always been able to achieve). The general structure of the meetings is that each person gets a chance to offer any personal or family "updates" about significant events that have happened since the last meeting. In the past, we also generally posed one or two questions around particular themes that had emerged in the research and put them to the group for discussion. With the permission of families, we have both audiotaped and videotaped these meetings. We have always served lots of food, and meetings take place during mealtimes.

Early in the development of these Collective Narrative Groups, Mary and I set a few basic ground rules to try to ensure that people would feel listened to and respected, despite the great diversity of those invited to the groups. The key "rules" (which Mary and I have announced ritually at the beginning of every meeting) are: everyone gets a chance to speak, there is no right answer, everyone has a right to his or her own opinions and experiences, people should feel free to show whatever emotions they want, and whatever is said in the group remains confidential in the sense that we will only report what is discussed using pseudonyms. It has dawned upon me that we unconsciously adopted rules that one might easily hear at any twelve-step meeting. While they may seem a bit jargonlike, they have seemed to work. Parents have told us that they have been able to say things in the group they were not even willing to tell their own family members; so perhaps there is something to say for this attempt to create some kind of safety. And oddly, people have sometimes decided to share much more personal parts of their lives in these meetings than they have in individual interviews, even when speaking to researchers they knew quite well. It is worth mentioning that some family members have become friends as a result of their years meeting up with us.

Discursive-Centered Ethnography

Given our commitment not to begin with a priori race, class, or economic determinisms, what has been perhaps the most surprising is the way this mode of ethnography has helped to illuminate the structural or discursive conditions that shape events and personal lives. Our micro-ethnographic approach, with its heavy reliance on the analysis of clinical and home interactions, has made it possible to analyze the workings not only of intimate personal or interpersonal dramas but also of the discursive genres of hope (which I will discuss in the following chapter) as practiced in very small, nearly invisible gestures. These genres, in their pervasiveness and global sweep, become visible not so much as abstract ideals but as the very stuff of everyday social interaction, pervading even the minute routines and dramas of ordinary life. The discursive, in other words, becomes visible as something intricately acted.

It has been important that we have conducted research within a variety of clinical spaces. This method of carrying out longitudinal and comparative institutional ethnography has allowed us to consider the role of particular kinds of institutional cultures in which health care takes place. Further, following children with a range of medical conditions has brought us into contact with many clinical subcultures in a given setting. This situatedness across several clinical sites (and clinical subcultures) has proven extremely helpful for an analysis of hope (especially clinical hope) at a discursive level. The "canonical" clinical genres of hope that I will describe in the next chapter are those that one can find variously expressed and acted across these institutional sites and clinical subspecialties.

Further, following families into their home and community spaces, and doing so across time, has also allowed us to track (from the inside, so to speak) how other structural conditions have impinged upon their lives: for example, such material matters as changes in the economy, in the demographics of housing and living patterns in Los Angeles, in the way health care is delivered, and in the way public funding for health care and welfare is allocated. While these do not form primary topics of this book, witnessing and documenting how families (and sometimes clinicians) struggle with changing laws and levels of economic support for health care reveals the structural as something immediately, often painfully, lived. Not surprisingly, the practice of hope—even hope for healing—is immensely influenced by these shifting political and economic conditions.

WHAT FOLLOWS: THE CHAPTERS

In this first chapter I have begun to sketch the main claims that will be elaborated throughout the book and have given some background about my own entrance into the clinical scene. I have also offered a space—both literal and metaphorical—that serves as my primary stage upon which to explore how dramas of hope unfold. Within this liminal space I have introduced Andrena, a central character in the book.

In the following chapter I plunge directly into a theoretical outline of narrative phenomenology. The framework I set out might be thought of as a kind of tool kit of narrative constructs with which to explore hope "dramatistically" both at the level of events and at the level of discursive structures. At the level of events, I demarcate three kinds of narrative acts: narrative mind reading, narrative emplotment, and storytelling. At the discursive level, I introduce four primary genres of healing that are in continual circulation in clinical encounters. These genres provide powerful cultural resources for clinicians and families, a social imaginary of hope in which hope is linked to healing. Three are clinically canonical: they offer plots that belong to, and dramatically express, authorized discourses of hope in the clinical world. In these clinic-centered dramas, the clinician, generally a physician, and disease itself are the primary characters. But the most important from the perspective of the families is a fourth genre: healing as transformative journey. In this one, unlike the first three, patients and families are the "main characters." Their lives, personal, familial, and communal, emerge as the critical sites in which hope and healing are to be fashioned.

While in chapter 2 I offer some small examples of clinical interchanges to help illustrate this tool kit of constructs, it is in the third chapter that the ethnography proper really opens. Turning again to Andrena, I begin an examination of the clinical encounter as a contested border space and as a space producing "familiar strangers" who are blamed for all manner of trouble. Here and in chapter 4, I take a close look at some highly charged moments where difficulties and misunderstandings arise between clinicians and parents. In these and the chapters that follow, I call upon the narrative acts and healing genres I outlined in the second chapter to examine how hope is contested, refused, negotiated, and created in the fragile and fraught partnerships between families and clinicians.

Having spent two chapters looking at the kinds of trouble that clinicians and parents can get into, and how easily hope is thwarted, I explore in chapters 5 and 6 the creation of hope in clinical encounters and how hope travels between clinic and home. Chapter 6 also investigates the role of an unexpected resource of hope: broadly circulated popular culture stories, Hollywood-marketed fantasies consumed by children. I look at how these "daydreams" are appropriated by children, clinicians, and family members as a means to explore possible worlds and identities that cannot be realized literally but can suggest new spaces for hope.

Chapter 7 examines why the practice of hope, even when cultivated and nurtured by clinicians, children, and parents, so easily falters. It explores the mystery of why clinicians so often seem not to recognize their own role in fostering hope for families and children even when they have become masterful at it. The concluding chapter (chapter 8) summarizes and extends some of the main claims of narrative phenom-enology and what it offers to an understanding of hope as a practice of creating communities in clinical borderlands. I end the book, however, not with abstract commentary but with a return (as perhaps befits an anthropological phenomenology) to the lives of two of the people I have written about. I offer something of an epilogue to consider what has happened to them since the clinical moments I described in earlier chapters.

CHAPTER 2

Narrative Matters

THE PRACTICE OF HOPE

What, precisely, does it mean to say hope is a practice? On the one hand, this seems obvious. For the past several decades, anthropology and the social sciences generally have shown an interest in practice. The term is now so ubiquitous it seems mere commonplace. What else could a culture, a social structure, or a local moral world be if not something somehow "practiced"? But of course, this construct has come into play because of a particular intellectual history. Aristotle made practice (or praxis) central to his political and ethical thought. Within social theory it has been most notably developed by Marx, who offered his famous dictum that human consciousness itself is shaped in and through activity. It continues to flourish as a key term in Marxist- (and Soviet-) inspired traditions.[1]

But the contemporary use of *practice* as an everyday term in social and cultural thought can be especially credited to poststructuralist theories of practice that the French in particular have given us: Pierre Bourdieu (1977, 1980, 1987; Bourdieu and Wacquant 1992), Michel Foucault (1965, 1995, 1973, 1979), and Michel de Certeau (1984). Anthony Giddens (1979, 1991), in England, and Marshall Sahlins (2000) and Sherry Ortner (2006), in the United States, have also been important early influences in shaping a "practice turn." Among them, Bourdieu may still stand as a central father figure, but Foucault's theory of discursive and regulatory practice offers the most creative, wide-ranging and influential view of the lot—a continuing inspiration for theorizing about the embodied and microscopic features of pervasive "regimes of truth."

While there is no single tradition of practice theory, some broadly shared problematics have engaged most of them and are pertinent for my purposes. Many practice theorists have taken up a set of concerns that have emerged particularly around the "structuration" of power. A primary question has concerned how everyday praxis leads to the perpetuation of social structures that not only are hierarchical but reproduce vast systems of immense political, cultural, and economic inequalities. Social practice theories inspired by Bourdieu have been concerned especially with the reproduction of certain distributions of cultural capital. All societies are built upon infrastructures that guarantee an unequal distribution of not only economic but also symbolic capital, as Bourdieu has taught us. Practices, the ways actors inhabit bodies and lived domains, their "habitus," reveal how this unequal distribution of power and wealth is invisibly reproduced. Everyday activities, the practice of the quotidian, unconsciously guarantee the continued existence of an unequal distribution of power.

Practice theorists have also been instrumental in promoting an examination of cultural life as materialized through the regulation of the body. Culture has come to be treated as less "in the head" than in the materiality of bodies in everyday action. Thus there is an emphasis on how social groups *do things* and how that doing is socially embodied, formative of personal and social identities, and central to the reproduction of social groups and discourse. For practice theorists, the body and subjectivity itself are constructed through relations of power. In an intellectual move that has proved extremely fruitful, theorists like Bourdieu and Foucault have offered ways to consider the body's subjectivity as *subjugation*. Phenomenology, here, is wedded to—or derivative of—the social structures or "regimes of truth" that dictate not merely highly visible social phenomena (the panoptic architectures of schools, hospitals, and prisons, for instance) or well-disguised social infrastructures (like nearly invisible flows of capital) but the micro bodily routines of everyday life.

Even when not explicitly acknowledged, the contemporary image of social worlds as border spaces that produce difference through insidiously diffused regulatory schemes ("structuring structures") owes a great deal to poststructuralist practice theorists. It is now part of anthropological and sociological common sense to excavate the underlying discursive practices that shape and govern bodies, temporalities, the very heart of experience for people "on the ground." Even as scholars work to consider social life as contested, dynamic, and hybrid (Abu-Lughod 2008), there is an increased tendency to see these contested moments as aspects of global diffusions of economic or neoliberal discursive power.

WHY WE NEED LIVED EXPERIENCE IN OUR PRACTICE THEORIES

This intellectual legacy means that it is difficult to speak of the practice of hope (or practice at all) without looking first and foremost at the structural conditions that underlie and regulate everyday activity and experience. But if we want, as I do, to examine hope as a practice that is "contested, dynamic, and hybrid," poststructuralist theories do not take us far enough. They easily obscure life on the ground in all its local and personal immediacy. Because so much attention has been directed to dominant structural activities (what de Certeau [1984] calls "strategies"), it has neglected those social activities invisible from this top-down vantage point (what de Certeau calls "tactics"). But less visible tactics are everywhere, and they too shape the spaces of action and possibility. They find their way into a host of "underground practices" of clinical work where hope is fostered by clinicians, parents, and children in a manner largely unacknowledged by them, by dominant biomedical discourse, or by social theorists of biomedicine. And even beneath the tactics de Certeau speaks of are the small dramas of ordinary life that cannot be captured by a practice theory that neglects the particularity of events and persons. Even when one is exploring hope as border work that is politically fraught, racially charged, and shaped by biomedicine's potent discursive practices, it is essential to be reminded of the way moments of possibility and community are cultivated and cherished across formidable divides.

Put in the bluntest terms: reality needs to be exposed as a space of possibility and not only of imprisonment or structural reproduction. Despite the immense power of oppressive social structures, reality is not summed up by their existence. It is not more real to disclose our imprisonment within everyday life than to disclose the possibilities for transformation that this life also admits. Ordinary people can and do still act, even in their ordinary contexts. They sometimes do struggle to remake lives in the most remarkably barren social circumstances. And sometimes these struggles make a difference.

Such critiques are not new. They have their own intellectual history, one that precedes poststructuralism itself but rests upon a long-standing tension between social accounts that emphasize large-scale social and political structures and accounts that emphasize lived experience and some form of personal agency. In fact, one of the most vexing problems for social theory has been precisely this: how to pay attention to large realities, the sorts so well suited to poststructuralist accounts, as well as the personal, intimate realities faced by on-the-ground people, the small realities that phenomenological projects have been committed to interpret. For several decades, the intellectual terrain has been primarily governed by structural (now poststructural, postcolonial, or postcritical) frameworks and phenomenological or experience-near ones. This division has provoked any number of debates over the years. It has not been an equal discussion either. Social theorists have been reluctant (as they have mostly always been reluctant) to *theoretically* privilege experience. Within anthropology, this lack of attention has also been evidenced in a lack of critical exploration of experience as a theoretical construct.[2] Only a minority of scholars have treated social life in explicitly phenomenological terms. An even smaller minority have attended to connections between the phenomenological and what, to borrow Arthur Kleinman's (2006) apt phrase, we might call "moral experience." These experience-minded minorities have been vocal. There have been protests. There have been justifications. But in general, the phenomenological trend has never caught on in a mainstream kind of way. On the whole, phenomenological accounts have been left trying to defend themselves, or to protest about what is "left out" of large-scale structural social pictures, by arguing for a concern with subjectivity that cannot be reduced to a subject position.

While the experience-centered tradition has a significant history, there is an almost disheartening similarity to the protests scholars working within this tradition have made to the various cultural, functional, structural, and now poststructural theories of their time. A. Irving Hallowell, using the vocabulary of his day and speaking of the experience-centered tradition in relation to cultural anthropology, put it this way: "The traditional approach of cultural anthropology . . . has been culture-centered, rather than behavior-centered" and has been organized through anthropologically conventional categories (1955:88). The problem with this, Hallowell asserts, is that such "cultural data do not easily permit us to apprehend, in an integral fashion, the most significant and meaningful aspects of the world of the individual as experienced by him and in terms of which he thinks is motivated to act, and satisfies his needs" (1955:88). We need, as D.T. Linger says many decades later, "a dialogue between those who wish to theorize about mind and persons without isolating them from society and history and those who wish to theorize about macrosocial phenomena without dehumanizing them" (1994:307). The idea that subjectivity is essentially epiphenomenal to social structures continues to marginalize the phenomenological.

The tenaciousness of this theoretical problem is perhaps also its gift. It has continued to provoke numerous creative attempts to bring together multiple analytic perspectives and include new ones (especially postcolonial and feminist theories) in ways that honor the phenomenological as well as the structural and that explore relationships between subjectivity and the political orders that help shape it. In the past decade, focusing upon sites of suffering and practices of healing, scholars have been attempting to develop new ways to speak about personal experience while at the same time exploring how subjectivities are shaped by the polities in which people dwell and by the social problems they endure.

In light of my own investigations of chronic illness among a group that continues to bear the mark of its colonial history, still subject to racial stigma, political violence, and economic suppression, the problem of how to integrate experience with large-scale political and social structures is worthy of special mention. The introduction of the term *social suffering* in the late 1990s has provided a framework around which some of this recent work has emerged. As discussed by Arthur Kleinman, Veena Das, and Margaret Lock (1997), we need to think of suffering as social and not merely personal (especially in cases of poverty or mass violence) because health problems are intertwined with political, economic, and institutional conditions, with the way power is structured and wielded.[3]

DRAMATIZING PRACTICE

What might a narrative phenomenology of practice have to offer a study of hope? How might it allow hope to be connected to social as well as personal suffering and to an understanding of healing as something both structural and intimate? Can a dramatistic practice theory help illuminate life as lived at multiple levels—in personal lives, inter-personal events, and discursive structures? Can it, in other words, teach us about hope and the creation of border communities in a way that allows us to see hope through the prisms of the personal and eventful as well as the structural? I will begin to answer these questions by broadly outlining what I mean by a narrative (or dramatistic) portrait of practice.

More than sixty years ago, Kenneth Burke (1945) proposed a frame-work of what he called "dramatism" for the study of social action and distinguished it from the leading theories of his time, which were based on behaviorist models. Behaviorism, he declared, was "designed to study people as mere things" (1966:53), needing no strong theory of agency and intention—of the centrality of *motive* to practical life and practical understanding. He offered an alternative theory in which motive, character, plot, scene—the terms we know from our under-standing of drama—could illuminate the complexity of action and com-munication. During this period, Victor Turner was developing a notion of social dramas that has continued to bear fruit in studies not only of ritual action but also of social life more generally. In the late 1960s, and for the next two decades, within philosophy of history, a debate took place that made narrative central to ideas of explanation of social action. Could one claim that history did not simply tell stories but in the telling also offered a particular mode of explanation—narrative explanation—that should be distinguished from the sorts of causal explanations that the physical sciences privileged (Dray 1993)? Within psychoanalysis as well, a new narrative understanding of therapeutic practices emerged. Perhaps what effective psychotherapy offered was a means to help patients retell their own life stories in new ways, a means to narratively reframe their lives, to tell a different sort of story about their past that might allow them to envision a different sort of story for their future (Schafer 1992).

In the 1980s, likely inspired by all these discussions, "narrative" burst upon the intellectual scene in a central way. Suddenly, and from several quarters, there arose a heightened interest in narrative in a way that extended far beyond its identification with storytelling. Clifford Geertz (1980) suggested that a "dramatistic turn" was occurring in the social sciences and linked it to his own highly literary interpretive anthropology. Most central for my purposes, *narrative* emerged as a key term with which to consider the temporality of lived experience; the self; moral action and ethics; suffering; and even the structure of thought itself.[4] Psychology, literary theory, philosophy, history, anthropology, sociology, medical humanities—each of these fields has had something to contribute to an understanding of social life and our experience of time as a narratively shaped unfolding of events. Dramatism, in its several guises, continues to flourish (though less visibly) in all these disciplines and in some cases has been suggestively brought into considerations of social practice.[5] It continues to occupy a central place within the medical humanities and medical ethics. Notably, "narrative medicine" is the name given to innovative attempts to train clinicians to be more "human centered" in their clinical care.

My own dramaturgical orientation builds upon much of this work.[6] I begin with this premise: as everyday actors, we locate ourselves in unfolding stories that inform our commitments about what is possible and desirable, our narrative anticipations and judgments about how things should and will unfold, and an understanding of the motives and actions of our interlocutors. In virtue of our participation within various "communities of practice" (Lave and Wenger 1991), we enter situations armed with narrative resources that prepare us to find our way in them. Practice is structural in the sense that it is prefigured by culturally specified plot structures that are expressed and dispersed throughout even the material infrastructure of a social world. These are not emotionally neutral or merely cognitive cultural schemas that are "in the heads" of participants but politically charged dramas that shape the rhythms of activity and the experiences and expectations of participants. They fill the social landscape with friends and enemies, with authorized desires and commitments, with identifiable members of one's community and outsiders. They people the landscape with social hierarchies. They are very often conflict driven, providing an anticipatory understanding of who has power and legitimacy to act in certain ways and under what circumstances, who are the keepers of truth, knowledge, and expertise, where risks lie, what is worth taking risks for, where trouble is likely to occur, and a number of other dramatic concerns.

The narrative framework I propose attends to a quality of social action often remarked upon by scholars of narrative texts. This is their ability to reveal life in time as something not predictable but rather, to follow Roland Barthes (1975), something plausible after all. The "after all" speaks volumes. It is a comment on the unexpectedness of events that unfold in narrative time, the contingent (it could have been otherwise) or even unfinished (suspenseful) quality of lived experience. As practical beings we are called to understand our situations in relation to an as yet unlived future. We are also called to contextualize our personal and social lives within a sense of the past. Practice evinces a complex temporal structure because it invokes a past (which in some way it continues even through its breaches and ruptures) and a future (which it moves toward, however indeterminately and suspensefully). Narrative (or drama) is such an important candidate for a theory of practice because it can challenge the hegemony of structural accounts precisely by highlighting the unfinished, idiosyncratic, unpredictable, suspenseful qualities of life. It can do so because it locates practice within the exigencies of human temporality and can reveal the contingencies of social life from multiple temporal perspectives, from small moments to broad cultural histories. The events and situations in which actors find themselves are also shaped by various histories, including the histories of those practices themselves. From such a perspective, events are moments, short stories within histories that are at once biographical, intimately interpersonal, and social in the broadest possible sense. Even our most intimate and personal practices reflect our human historicity, our situatedness in social time.[7] As Gadamer put it, "The great historical realities of society and state always have a predeterminant influence on any 'experience'" (1975:245), so no model of understanding practical action can rest with personal or subjective experience alone.[8]

It should be very evident that within the dramatistic tradition and the narrative phenomenology I am proposing, the term *narrative* is not used in its ordinary sense. While in common parlance when we speak of narrative we have in mind either a kind of artifact (a text) or a genre of speech act, for my purposes this framework is not large enough and is in many ways misleading, seeming to dissolve the embodied and the practical into the linguistic. Storytelling and the reception of cultural texts represent one small part of how narrative infuses practical action and lived experience.[9] It is in part to underscore this expansion of "narrative" that I link it so closely to "drama." In drawing from multiple disciplines, I use the closely interlinked terms *drama* and *narrative* almost interchangeably. This is not intended to contribute to terminological confusion; rather, I wish to highlight how each of these terms brings with it a scholarly history that is helpful in outlining a narrative phenomenology of practice. I interweave my use of them to invoke these intellectual histories as well as to point to some general and interconnected features of social practice that make these kindred terms. Drama is perhaps the most obvious frame to use in order to underscore a primary focus upon the eventfulness *of social action* rather than its textual representation or the performance of speech genres. The term *narrative* invokes other, equally useful intellectual traditions, including hermeneutic phenomenology with its considerations of the temporal complexity of practical time as well as moral philosophy in which narrative has been connected to the cultivation of a moral self.

THE MULTIPLE LEVELS OF PRACTICE: WRITING AGAINST STRUCTURE

In the remainder of this chapter, I sketch a narrative portrait of practical action that encompasses an experience-near level of analysis (populated by persons, events, and encounters) and, in addition, those sorts of macro phenomena—large-scale cultural, historical, and social formations—visible only from a certain more distant analytic position. I will thus try to offer a theory of practice that illuminates life as lived at multiple levels, and in a way that does not collapse any one level into another, thereby turning everything into the "mere expression" of a single line of sight.

I seek to "write against structure" in the sense of offering an alternative vision to structural determinisms that make personal lives and small events mere epiphenomena, the local results of global forces and discursive practices. The task is how to consider the structural not only as large cultural and historical narratives that shape everyday interaction but also from a dramatistic perspective that subverts a portrait of them as totalizing narrative frames.

I turn to Kenneth Burke to help illuminate this. Speaking of literary dramas, he offers the following comments about how the structural, which he refers to (dramatistically) as the "scene," operates. For him, the structural is not simply an abstraction that subsumes particular characters and their actions. Nor is it located high above the heads (or below the ground) of individuals and their predicaments. Rather, the scene functions as one of the major vehicles through which drama is produced. It has direct dramatic force as one among many key elements that influence the course of events. In fiction, Burke notes, "it is a principle of drama that the nature of acts and agents should be consistent with the nature of the scene" (1945:3). However, this principle of consistency is the very thing that is regularly violated for dramatic effect. A dramatic moment commonly involves agents acting in ways that are at odds with the scene, generating all sorts of Trouble that must then be resolved in some fashion. Thus (in the world of fictional stories) the scene is not in some untouchable way outside the drama of human interaction. It, too, can be manipulated and transformed. While the scene is in one sense a backdrop or container, it can be shifted by the elements (agents, their actions) contained. And it is, in fact, the destabilizing of relationships between container and contained (often resulting in transformations of both) that triggers a dramatic moment.[10]

In general, social theories dealing with a nonfictitious world of "real life" represent the scene as quite beyond the reach of agents and their acts. The scene emerges as an overwhelmingly powerful container (cultural, political, economic, etc.) that explains why individuals in particular situations behave as they do. Such an explanatory strategy is the ruin of fiction because it defeats the possibility of drama and, if you follow Burke, the possibility of action at all, at least action anyone could care about. In works of fiction, he notes, too much consistency between container and contained will undermine the plot itself. Burke gives the example of the unfortunate storyteller who runs into this very problem: "He may choose to 'indict' some scene (such as bad working conditions under capitalism) by showing that it has a 'brutalizing' effect upon the people who are indigenous to this scene. But the scene-agent ratio, if strictly observed here, would require that the 'brutalizing' situation contain 'brutalized' characters as its dialectical counterpart. And thereby, in his humanitarian zeal to save mankind, the novelist portrays characters which, in being as brutal as their scene, are not worth saving" (1945:9).

In social theories where the "scene" is overwhelmingly dictatorial, the agents contained within it can only mirror its characteristics in their actions and dispositions, or, as we say in anthropology, "internalize" and "reproduce" the external social conditions in their own docile bodies. It is precisely this problem of docility that needs to be redressed in our social theories, even while we foreground the oppressive qualities of social structures. How to clear some space for action? How to give us characters we can care about, ones who are not merely puppets or victims of their social conditions?

Here is my approach. Rather than foregrounding a habitus, social structure, or regime of truth as a kind of collective container of practical agents and practical action, in the ethnographic chapters that follow I focus primarily upon the agents themselves, on the ground and in their particularity, examining their efforts in situational and personal detail, treating these larger macrostructures as powerful cultural resources (including highly negative resources) that inform but do not determine their actions, their experiences, and their deliberations. This means that I am *not* making certain kinds of questions central to my analysis in the way that they are for poststructuralist practice theory and, more broadly, for contemporary anthropology generally. I certainly call upon large-scale social categories that fall under names like race, class, gender, religion, disability, and biomedicine, and there are a variety of instances throughout this book in which parents, children, and clinicians are represented as reproducing, resisting, or working to amend these social categories. I very often try to analyze how this happens. However, I am not, to put it briefly, most concerned about the social life of categories. Rather, my investigation is more phenomenological, more person-centered, precisely because I attend to how these categories help to shape and inform the hopes that people bring to illness, suffering, and healing, making that practical problem, which is of such consuming interest to the families I write about, the central focal point. It is in this strong sense that I treat social categories as cultural resources that inform life on the ground, not as containers that enclose it.

EVENT-CENTERED PRACTICE

If we begin with actors located in situations not necessarily of their own choosing, and with a complex and only partially conscious arrays of motives, actors who are also attempting to shape those situations and discern what is "worth hoping for" in them, the drama of practice quickly becomes evident. Situations also reveal how social life is much more than the purely personal and explicitly intentional. Attention to events "illuminates what is at stake for those involved" but also directs us to "ethical and practical implications that far outrun specific individual intentions and awareness" (Jackson 2005:75).

The events I depict throughout this book highlight the way actors endlessly try to ascertain what is in the minds and hearts of themselves and others and try to transform the motives, emotions, and actions of themselves and others. This is also very much a *person-centered* picture of practice because it puts human action, motives, and foibles at the center. I will offer a picture of persons in connection with other persons trying to read minds, tell stories, and create experiences. These intimate interpersonal "we's" and these social exchanges also presume biographical "I's." Of course, the personal is dependent upon the sociality of practice and experience, and any "I" is necessarily constructed within a social history, in the midst of living a social life. Yet the personal is indispensable analytically, and it is deeply implicated in the way I analyze the narrative qualities of social interactions and events. The dramas that are created through social interactions and in social contexts carry not only social meanings but personal ones as well. And these matter. The event in which Andrena first hears about her daughter's cancer, for example, is not only a social event—it is an event for Andrena, an event that changes her life. Events take their meaningful shape (are lived experiences) for actors depending upon what they bring to the encounter and what is at stake for them personally.

At the event-centered level, I will speak of practice in terms of a closely interlinked set of narrative acts: "narrative mind reading," "narrative emplotment," and "storytelling." These narrative activities are rooted in particular social histories and take their particular cultural shape from those histories. They also reveal the micro activities of everyday life and how these challenge, improvise upon, and sometimes creatively reinvent or play with those histories. I describe them briefly below. While it is useful to separate these narrative activities for analytic purposes, in actual situations they are inevitably intertwined. When they are placed in ethnographic context, as they are in subsequent chapters, their interdependency will become obvious.

Narrative Mind Reading: The Narrativity of Practical Action

The notion of "narrative mind reading" speaks most obviously to the infusion of narrative reasoning into practical action. Because we are predisposed to apprehend the world in narrative terms, we bring what one might call *narrative preunderstandings* to action.[11] One aspect of our narrative preunderstanding involves our continuous ascription of motives to the actions of those around us, such that we "read" intentionality from their observable behavior in terms of our understanding of the context. *Narrative mind reading,* as I am using this term, concerns the linking of what someone does—his or her observable actions—to a motive. It is an investigation of an interior landscape by way of an exterior one. Motive becomes central. Generally this is not a consciously deliberative process but an automatic one—we simply *see* a smile or a grimace or a sneer (however much the facial expression may be similar) when we look at someone's face.

It has long been recognized that even the names used to describe human actions involve claims about intentions. That is, assigning names to human acts, including the simplest ones, requires such discernment. The philosopher Gilbert Ryle uses the example of twitches (involuntary) and winks (motivated): the same observable behavior but two different acts. Geertz (1973) famously drew on Ryle's example to speak of the work that culture does in allowing members of a social group to distinguish twitches from winks, or burlesques of winks, et cetera. But as Alasdair MacIntyre adds, these ascriptions require something more than general cultural knowledge. To know what someone is doing we have to place it in a context that makes the action intelligible to us, and this context is, above all, a narrative one. "An action," he writes, "is a moment in a possible or actual history or in a number of such histories" (1981:199). For an action to be intelligible at all, we must place it within some sort of "possible or actual history." We see it as an episode in a story. Paul Ricoeur gives a supporting argument that suggests why narrative is so basic to our understanding of action. He contends that actions belong to a "network" that includes goals, motives, and agents who can be held responsible. All these must be connected in the everyday synthetic work of practical understanding. "Actions imply goals, the anticipation of which is not to be confused with some foreseen or predicted result, but which connect the one on whom the action depends. Actions, moreover, refer to motives, which explain why someone does or did something. . . . Actions also have agents, who do and can do things which are taken as their work, their deed. As a result, these agents can be held responsible for certain consequences of their actions" (1984:55). And since narratives (as texts) also connect actions to goals, motives, agents, and consequences, it makes sense, Ricoeur concludes, to consider action as having a "proto-narrative" form. The ascription of motive to practical action is so centrally bound up with a narrative form of cognition that Jerome Bruner (1986, 1990) has made a compelling case that this narrative form of reasoning constitutes one of two basic forms of human thought and underlies a culture's "folk psychology."

This narrative work is socially rooted. We are capable of narrative apprehension in particular situations because of our culturally shaped narrative expectations. Our cultural knowledge gives us the resources to construct stories in which others' actions, and our own, can be understood as meaningful contributions to unfolding plots. Cultures provide resources for action because they allow us to invent plausible narrative scenarios and help us to place our own actions and those of others within possible histories. They supply us with the ability to construct or envision stories that we and others are living out. It is these imagined unfolding stories that allow us to see given actions as actions of a particular sort. They also offer us forward momentum, shaping our commitments and our dramatic reading of potential troubles, risks, enemies, allies, and the like. To quote Jerome Bruner on the matter: "When we enter human life, it is as if we walk on stage into a play whose enactment is already in progress—a play whose somewhat open plot determines what parts we may play and toward what denouements we may be heading" (1990:34).

In the final part of this chapter where I attend to the discursive level of practice, I will have much more to say about this social or cultural dimension of mind reading as it plays out in the clinical world. But to give a small illustration here, I recall Andrena's account of hearing the news that her daughter was gravely ill. She remembers that the doctor began by saying, "I'm so sorry." These chilling words sent Andrena into a complete panic. "So sorry?" Andrena replied. "Did you hear something else?" Andrena had no difficulty recognizing that "sorry" in this context was not an apology for wrongdoing on the physician's part but a moment of empathy for the news that she was about to hear. Her instant sense of dread signaled that she knew the cultural context well enough (she had been taken aside into a small room away from the waiting room) that this "sorry" announced that she had found herself in an illness story that was only going to get worse. And she was absolutely right.

It makes sense to claim that at some moments knowing what someone is doing (e.g., distinguishing whether in saying "I'm sorry" someone is apologizing or offering sympathy) does not require an investigation into the mysteries of someone else's mind, only an understanding of the social context, a more or less public assessment of behavior. But this picture of culturally mediated mind reading is complicated if one sees "culture" not as a stable system of reference that allows individuals who "live in it" to discern what others are up to but as a border zone of conflicting messages and references. Narrative mind reading emerges as a critical aspect of the practical problem of creating partnerships with "foreigners" in order to get one's job done.

Unsurprisingly, in a borderland like the hospital Andrena found herself in, mind reading is often a source of misunderstanding. There is often a pervasiveness of mind *misreading* in clinical encounters that obstructs the social construction of hope between families and clinicians. In the cultural space of the clinic, preunderstandings are very often misunderstandings. For the African American families in our study, the question of race became intimately bound up with such mind reading. There would be times when Andrena would wonder whether a physician's statement like "I'm so sorry" also conveyed a different sort of apology, one indicating that because she was black and on public aid, her daughter was not getting the same quality of treatment that a white and "private pay" child would receive.

Narrative Emplotment: The Social Dramas of Everyday Life

If all social action has a fundamentally narrative character because mind reading relies upon narrative preunderstandings, some moments are "more narrative than others" (Mattingly 1998a:129). Lived time is uneven. There emerge certain moments, events, and encounters that, as we commonly say, are "dramatic" or "memorable" as opposed to "routine" or "forgettable." Sometimes more narrative moments are likely to be remembered in stories we later tell, as when Andrena narrates her experience getting the diagnosis for her daughter. When the doctor told Andrena, "I'm so sorry," this was part of a moment that sliced Andrena's life into two. It reshaped her life into a new one; it demarcated a "before" and an "after." The dramatic import (from mundane to highly significant) of any present moment for any particular actor depends upon how it is situated between remembered (and unremembered) pasts and anticipated futures within multiple kinds and levels of histories—from the most global to the most intimately personal.[12]

These "more narrative" moments may be precipitated by outside events (like the sudden onslaught of an illness), but they are not merely received. They are acted upon. To emphasize this productive aspect of significant experience, I speak about narrative *emplotment*. In the first chapter I mentioned my earlier work where, with an eye to one type of emplotment, I wrote about "healing dramas." Healing dramas open up a world of possibilities, allowing participants to inhabit "as if" worlds that have transformative, sometimes even socially radical, implications for becoming. In this book, I especially examine clinical moments where hope particularly resides in the cultural work of creating common ground among clinicians and family members. Such dramas offer moments of *social* healing that speak to social divides created by race, class, and disabling illness. These moments may be fleeting and fragile, but when they arise their achievement is very often marked (at least by families) as deeply significant.

But of course, conflictual dramas also arise in clinical encounters. Clinicians and families inadvertently get in one another's way even while attempting to enact healing plots. Conflict dramas set rhythms of opposition into motion, generating skirmishes that prevent others from realizing possibilities or hopes and intensifying misunderstandings among participants. These dramatic moments offer a phenomenological window into misunderstanding as a lived experience, something that is not merely given by prior subject positions and cultural categories but acted. The conflict dramas I describe also illuminate in a particularly stark way how social and racial inequities are produced in the daily practices of clinical work. Conflicts can become episodes in unfolding dramas of disrespect and dismissal, arising even when all the actors share a deeply felt concern about the ill child.

Storytelling

Stories are everywhere in the hospital, and they are everywhere at home as parents care for their ill or disabled children. Stories are also agentive. They act in and on the world.[13] Stories can have powerful consequences upon how the present is experienced and what future actions seem most reasonable, likely, or appropriate. Storytelling "refigures" events into oral and written texts, and these texts—always performed—may circulate widely in social communities, influencing further actions. In this patent respect, stories about the past have enormous influence in shaping how the future is envisioned. Stories take their meaning not only from their content but also from the situation in which they are performed, including who is doing the telling.[14] Like other acts, they are tailored to context—in particular, the audience. Also, it is reasonable to speak of stories, like other social acts, as multiply authored in the sense that who listens powerfully shapes what is told and how it is interpreted. In reflective moments, stories can highlight the negotiated, situated, and interpreted quality of social life. They can even foreground a recognition that others, operating from another perspective, could tell a different story. In less reflective moments, stories can be compelling precisely because they *disguise* other interpretive possibilities. Seductive stories—stories that persuade—can offer powerful renditions of the "facts of the matter" concerning who did what to whom and what the consequences were.

While much has been written about storytelling in the clinical world, in this book I focus primarily on two of its many practical purposes. One is the way storytelling offers a vehicle (often unacknowledged) for making moral judgments through the configuring of the plot. Narratives can allow parents, patients, and clinicians to reason about what to do on the basis of what has occurred (as events are rendered through the story), who is to blame, who is responsible, who the characters are, what can be hoped for, and the like. Storytelling can play a powerful role in shaping moral judgments of narrators and audiences because stories' dramatic qualities rest on the exposure of a breach from the expected. They provide means for explaining why things have gone in a problematic or surprising direction; they simultaneously depict a version of the culturally appropriate and departures from it (Garro 2000, 2003). And they do so by presenting an unfolding series of events as they happen over time—in process rather than as completed facts or abstract propositions.

A second role of storytelling that I explore is the way that stories offer a picture of life as "subjunctive." Stories tell us about life that is inevitably *in the middle,* about an unfolding present that is always situated between past and future. The in-the-middle-ness of lived experience takes on an existential primacy in stories, as the novelist E. M. Forster notes. "Let us think of people," he recommends, "as starting life with an experience they forget and ending it with one which they anticipate but cannot understand" (1927:48). Andrena and other parents in our study also use stories to reflect on their own lives from this in the middle, liminal perspective. They or their children may even draw upon cultural stories that seem far removed from their daily experience as a way of introducing a liminal or "what if" perspective, reimagining who they are and who they are becoming.[15]

DRAMATIZING STRUCTURE: DISCURSIVE-CENTERED PRACTICE

Hope is *discursively centered* in cultural genres that shape its cultivation and suppression within particular cultural contexts. Within the clinical context are a set of powerful dramatic plot structures that powerfully shape the healing practice of clinicians, families, and children whom I write about and that have immense salience in the popular culture of the United States. From the clinical point of view, three genres are particularly central: (1) healing as sleuthing; (2) healing as battling disease; and (3) healing as repairing broken machine-bodies. These canonical genres are also deeply embedded in the physical and social gestures of the clinic world. They offer idealized "happy endings" that embody, narratively, the ideals associated with biomedicine as an applied science—including prediction, control, clarity of goals, accumulation of knowledge, empirically tested methods, and standardized practices of reasoning. Taken together, they constitute a narrative infrastructure that offers a rich cultural resource through which minds are read, actions are emplotted, stories are told, and futures are envisioned. While families also rely upon these genres to make sense and act for the care of their child's illness or disability, for them another genre emerges as primary: (4) healing as transformative journey.

Healing genres are both performed and embodied; they are subtly invoked in myriad ways in clinical life, underlying the everyday organization of space, time, and bodies. Actors negotiate, interpret, understand, and misunderstand one another in light of them. In the context of providing health care in multicultural urban America, coming to some kind of mutual understanding about what parts may be played or even about *which* genre best fits the situation can be tricky business indeed.

Dominant healing genres in biomedicine provide an authorized action framework; they lay the ground of narrative—and normative—expectations for how things *should* unfold. At the core of these healing genres are highly evocative images or metaphors—tropes that suggest entire plot structures and characters, including villains and allies, heroes and helpmates. Ricoeur (1984) has argued all narratives are "extended metaphors." A narrative offers a figurative framing that "always means more than it literally says, says something other than what it seems to mean, and reveals something about the world only at the cost of concealing something else" (White 1999:7). The narrative's aesthetic structure is enormously important in determining what is attended to, what counts as evidence, how "facts" are constituted, and what is concealed. Not only do canonical narratives refuse certain practical realities that impinge upon clinical care (like race, class, and power), but they also obscure the intransigence and incurability of many clinical conditions. They are challenged by chronic disease, which thwarts their idealized happy endings.[16]

One of the most significant features of these canonical genres is that they are utopian. They have the potential to fuel imagination about possible, as yet unrealized futures, the undiscovered promise of science—a shadowy narrative horizon only hinted at by the realities of day-to-day clinical work. At the everyday level of clinical practice, the utopian power of medicine's canonical genres is not located solely in what any particular clinician can do or offer to her particular patients. Rather, their symbolic power rests within a more far-reaching drama of clinical hope that is part of the very development of modern biomedicine, what M. J. Good has called a "medical imaginary" (2007). This imaginary spans popular and professional cultures, is globally circulated, and offers a sense of possibility to research scientists, clinicians, and patients alike.[17]

The Canonical Genres

An idea of hope based upon scientific progress—and an instrumentally applied use of science to improve health and life—is an old story, of course. The utopian qualities of canonical plots are very much grounded in a hope based on scientific knowledge and technologies and the individual expertise of the clinician to deploy them. They are even grounded in hopes that clinicians and families have about what future biotechnologies may offer to these children and about new forms of biosociality that may further these possibilities.

The dark side of this utopian hope has been repeatedly exposed. Western biomedicine has been deeply implicated in the social aspirations of liberal and humanist projects of modernity. The history of modern medicine has gone hand in hand with the development of a particular notion of rationality, grounded (metaphorically as much as anything) in the vivid image of the doctor scientist. Medicine has accrued symbolic capital because of its presumptions about what constitutes knowledge and how truths are discovered. It draws its prestige and claim to truth by its relation to science. As an applied science that deals with the body, it "is interposed between formal science—our special source of 'truth' about natural processes—and the everyday experiences of such processes" (Comaroff 1982:55). Scientific experimentation is justified through "the production of scientific knowledge and its practices" and the "legitimization of such knowledge as truth" (Lock 1997:238).

The rise of modern medicine is often seen as a potent exemplar of hope gone wrong, especially the hope of a scientifically grounded rationality that could change the world. Foucault's studies of modern regimes of care have been a key source of inspiration. He has offered a sustained and inspired meditation on the failures and flaws of medicine's utopian hopes. At its darkest, Foucault's well-known dystopic histories offer portraits of the clinic as a kind of prison in which patients are guarded, disciplined, examined, and punished. His use of Bentham's great panoptic towers—the utopian vision of the modern prison—captures in a single image an entire societal drama of the gradual, disciplinary overtaking of all social structures and of the bodies that inhabit them, all in the name of reform.

One of Foucault's most interesting points is that this modern form of imprisonment grew out of an attempt to realize a grand social hope that linked new practices to new hopes about rationality itself. Foucault tells a story in which, after the French Revolution, medicine was imagined as a successor to the church. Medicine's dream was not only to replace the church but to help eradicate poverty itself. When poverty was abolished, this would be the end of sickness and of the hospitals in which the sick were housed. "No more indigents, no more hospitals" was one political battle cry. Even when this wildly optimistic dream had to be relinquished, a specious utopianism clung to ideals about clinical care and still reigns in myths of modern medicine, Foucault argues. This false hope is based upon the myth of no myths, the possibility of cultivating a neutral, clear gaze that can simply see what exists without illusion. This myth belongs to a utopian story of the march of science and the accumulation of knowledge.[18]

I now turn more specifically to the three canonical genres, drawing upon small examples from this research to illustrate how they operate in day-to-day clinic life. These examples will certainly illustrate some of their most troublesome and dystopic qualities, but they will also quickly complicate any idealized version of the canonical in either its negative or positive forms. Life on the ground—that is, at the level of events—is inevitably messier, or, as I would like to put it, more "dramatistic." It will come as no surprise that in practice the idealized qualities of these plot structures also become evident as they are modified, revised, or even largely discarded because of the exigencies of particular circumstances. Everyday clinical practice thus invokes and relies upon but also challenges the canonical genre's "mythic" claims to a neutrally defined truth, to the expert as purveyor of truth, and to their power to deliver "happy endings."

Healing as a Science Detective Story

This genre draws upon an image of medicine as an investigative, practical science. The key protagonists of this drama are the doctor (a Sherlock Holmes figure) and the disease itself, the mysterious culprit of medical crimes. The clinician as sleuth has the task of investigating medical mysteries, identifying the (hidden) criminal who perpetrates crimes inside a patient's body, leaving traces in the form of symptoms and signs that present puzzles to be deciphered. The analogy between the detective story and this image of clinical care is no accident. The medical case as a narrative form actually developed alongside the detective story as a literary form. While it might seem that medicine borrowed this narrative from literature, the relationship is more complex. Arthur Conan Doyle, who gave us Sherlock Holmes, was himself a physician, and the figure of Holmes was inspired by a famous physician teacher of the time, Dr. Bell, "a wizard of 'deduction' whose feats of clinical reasoning were legendary" (Hunter 1991:22).[19]

The detective story plays an especially critical role in case presentations. A medical mystery does not merely present itself as an empirical reality to the clinician but must be constructed. Learning to craft a medical mystery is an essential part of the skill that medical students need to master. Medical students learn to "build mystery into a clinical story" as a part of developing and exercising analytical abilities and clinical reasoning (M. Good 1995:137). The capacity to take a clinical case and make of it a medical mystery is part of the "persuasive craft" of the clinician and is directly tied to the clinician's ability to work with a medical team and influence the kinds of therapeutic decisions that are made (M. Good 1995:140).

In this focus upon the clinician and the disease, patients and family members are often left to one side—the drama can be extremely clinician centered, and the hierarchy of clinical command is often easily evident. Here is an instance not at all uncommon, speaking not only to the genre of detective story but also to another key canonical genre: repairing a broken machine. Dr. Parkman, a senior orthopedist at one of our clinical sites, brings in a group of residents to one of the physical therapy treatment rooms. He is going to examine Vernon, a six-year-old boy who has come with his grandmother, Effie, for his twice-weekly physical therapy session. Vernon was born with a congenital hip problem that requires an intensive home and outpatient physical therapy program; if the program is not successful, he will need surgery. While he and his grandmother see their physical therapist regularly, the visit by the orthopedist and residents is unexpected.

When these clinicians enter the small therapy room, the orthopedist quickly takes charge, interrupting the therapy session. The physical therapist stands back, allowing the physician to assume center stage, and assists in getting measures of range of motion and extension of Vernon's hips and legs. The residents form a respectful backdrop to the exchange between physician and therapist and the physician's examination of Vernon. Vernon and his grandmother, who are normally chatty during physical therapy sessions, fall completely silent. Although there is no grand "medical mystery" to solve (the clinicians know what the problem is), ongoing detective work is needed to determine how well the hip is improving with therapy as Vernon grows and if any other interventions (especially surgery) will be required. At the instruction of Dr. Parkman, a resident reads aloud off the medical chart: "Vernon is a six-year-old boy going to PT [physical therapy], where he performs range-of-motion exercises." Dr. Parkman then turns his attention to the physical therapist.

> Dr. Parkman: Range?
>
> Physical therapist: Abduction-wise, inflection 110, both bilateral.
>
> Dr. Parkman: What about . . .
>
> Physical therapist: (finishes) Measuring abduction and extension?
>
> Dr. Parkman: What's extension?
>
> Physical therapist: Last time it was about 45.

Upon hearing this news, the physician turns and addresses Vernon.

> Dr. Parkman: Not good, buddy. We might have to do surgery.

After this terrifying remark, the physical therapist hastily intervenes, noting that she hasn't done any measures that day. Dr. Parkman directs Vernon to hop up on a table where he can be examined. Vernon, still silent, does as he is told. The physician begins his examination, asking the therapist to supply information as he moves the child's legs up and down. He directs his findings and remarks primarily to the residents who surround him.

> Dr. Parkman: Get up here (indicating the table) and let me take a look.
>
> Physical therapist: Do you [want me to] measure arc?

Dr. Parkman: Yeah.

Physical therapist: (doing so) About 30–32 on left.

Dr. Parkman: (moves the boy's legs up and down) Not terrible. He's got the rotation.

Physical therapist: (referring to the home therapy program that Vernon is instructed to do) They've been really good about doing their exercises.

Dr. Parkman: (speaking to residents) It appears his hip is doing okay. It's in the healing phase. He has reasonable range of motion. So chances of having to do an operation are pretty small. The head of his leg bone may be getting too big for the socket. If that stabilizes we're okay. If not we're going to need the operation to maintain it. The goals are to (1) maintain rotation and (2) maintain the socket. His youth should help the healing process, but not everybody acts as he should. *(turning for the second time to address Vernon directly)* Still, no running or jumping.

While the neglect to bring patients or family caregivers into the clinical encounter that Dr. Parkman demonstrates is a common occurrence, often this is not the case. When it comes to the ongoing treatment of children's chronic conditions, detective work often depends upon partnerships created between clinicians and family caregivers; clinicians and family members are well aware of this. Clinicians will routinely judge when they have parents who can help them in their detective work. For example, Dr. Clark, an endocrinologist, described how important parents can be in assisting the diagnostic process. It is also clear from the small story he tells to make his point that he is working to train residents to learn how much parents can contribute to the job of detecting disease even if they are "not highly educated":

I just had a kid in clinic on Friday when I had a student with me, and this mom sat down. And she was a Spanish mom. She's pretty damn smart, but, you know, she's not a highly educated lady. And she was paying very careful attention to what happened to her kid when he was in intensive care. She basically described to me all of the medical history required to make a diagnosis of adrenal insufficiency. I remember, I said this to the student that was with me, I said, "You know, this mom described this, that's how we know." The student's like, "How do you know the kid's got Addison's disease?" I said, "Because the mom described the entire thing to me and I listened to her."

In fact, clinicians often work to train parents to collect information at home that can help them to pinpoint causes of a child's symptoms, actively requesting that they assist in the detective work. We can see this in the following exchange between a physician, Dr. Robbin, and

Leanna, the great-aunt of Matthew, a severely physically devastated child who has cerebral palsy. She has assumed the job of primary parent since the death of Matthew's mother and grandmother and the absence of his father. Dr. Robbin recruits Leanna to help in trying to determine what is triggering Matthew's unexpected seizures. According to Leanna, who is an extremely attentive parent, these seem to be precipitated by a "tickling sensation" in his throat. Although Matthew cannot speak in ordinary words, he is not, Leanna insists, uncommunicative. He has many means of making his wishes and desires known. Through the years of caring for him she has acquired knowledge of how to follow his language, which she very much considers a form of speech. (This will be seen in the conversation she has with Dr. Robbin where she tells him that Matthew "usually says when it itches" although that "saying" turns out to mean that he rubs under his jaw to indicate this itching.) She has a daily proximity to Matthew but also skills that Dr. Robbin lacks, which position her to gather needed information that could be pertinent to discovering the mysterious culprit of these seizures. She also has become adept enough at learning the language of biomedicine to follow Dr. Robbin's instructions to "stimulate his parotid" to see if this triggers the tingling in Matthew's throat. This could be a key sign that the seizures are food related.

> *Dr. Robbin:* Let's try, have you tried, when it happens, when he has that sensation, have you tried making a list of things that he ate at that particular time?
>
> *Leanna:* No, I haven't done that.
>
> *Dr. Robbin:* Um, why don't we try to keep a record . . .
>
> *Leanna:* Okay.
>
> *Dr. Robbin:* Write the date, okay, and write down everything that he ate at the particular meal at the time that you notice that.
>
> *Leanna:* Right.
>
> *Dr. Robbin:* And then keep your list at a place where you know where it is, like on the refrigerator or something, [and when it] happens again, write the date, make another list, and after about two or three times, see if you notice the same things showing up. That's one way we can do it.
>
> *Leanna:* Okay.
>
> *Dr. Robbin:* If it's possible, maybe [what] you can do . . . is if you stimulate his parotid you'll get a tingling sensation.
>
> *Leanna:* Yeah, 'cause he usually says that it itches.
>
> *Dr. Robbin:* Yeah, yeah.

Leanna: He's always . . . , he would do like this (*rubbing under her jaw*) afterwards.

Dr. Robbin: I mean, I remember when he was younger, he used to drool all the time.

Leanna: Yes.

Dr. Robbin: You know, so, maybe there's something going on with the salivary glands that are contributing to that itchy feeling. So, if we could pinpoint something that's triggering it off, then that's one approach.

But the mutual dependence of clinicians and families to create detective partnerships also has many pitfalls. As clinicians sometimes report, parents can create new kinds of problems. Inexperienced clinicians, a hematologist explains, can "scare" parents by delivering news about potential highly serious medical conditions that their child may have, thus producing "hypervigilant" parents who do not know how to report information properly. This can greatly confound the ongoing detective work that is so endemic to serious, chronic illnesses. Such "overvigilant" parents can contribute to the medical problems a child faces and make it much more difficult for physicians to analyze them properly.

If clinicians worry about parents who are hypervigilant or do not know how to report symptoms accurately, parents have their own anxieties. Many believe clinicians may simply refuse to do the proper sleuthing necessary to get to the bottom of their child's problem. They speak of their own need to learn to push back, especially with physicians, and to be willing to stand up to them rather than simply accepting their authority. Parents frequently tell stories about the misery of having to learn that they cannot simply rely on their child's doctors to be good detectives. Effective border crossing, in other words, is often precipitated by the painful realization that compliance is not the answer. Sandra, for example, describes how she learned to demand better investigative care for her child from her own mother, who was a nurse. A few months after Sandra's first child was born, her mother suspected that he was not developing properly. She became furious that Sandra's pediatrician (who was near retirement) was missing obvious cues of serious cognitive delay. She tried to get Sandra to confront him. Sandra did not want to. Her mother asked her: "Who is this old man? Is he asking you this? Is he asking you that?" When her mother confronted her, Sandra "would get upset with her." She remembers their arguments. "They know what they're doing," she would tell her mother. "Stop it, stop it, stop it!" But her mother persisted, and finally, when her son was four months old, they went to see the pediatrician together. Here is the scene she describes:

> He said [to her mother], "Oh Granny, he's a premie and this is something they go through." He just was like, "Oh, they take longer to do things, and you just gotta relax." And she says, "Listen, I'm a nurse and I've dealt with people like you. Sometimes you gotta just pay attention to the signs. And I don't know if you're stupid or if you're smart, but I know one thing. You're going to pay attention to this baby because I'm going to find the best lawyer that I can find or take my daughter out of this pediatrician's office." And I'm sitting there in shock that she's talking to him this way. And then he calmed down and said, "I'm sorry, I apologize. You're right. We'll insist that he goes to a specialist and make sure there's no harm, because he's not tracking. You're right."

The pediatrician finally made referrals to specialists. And this is how Sandra ended up getting a diagnosis of cerebral palsy for her son.

Healing as a Battle

In this culturally familiar genre, protagonists fight "the war against disease." In its canonical version, the clinicians and the disease are again the main characters. Pathology is a foreign invader that the physician and fellow clinicians must battle, and the patient's body is a "site" or "field" of the battle. This image also arose in the nineteenth century, though it has gone through several permutations as understandings of the body and its immune system have changed: "The military metaphor in medicine first came into wide use in the 1880s, with the identification of bacteria as agents of disease. . . . Bacteria were said to 'invade' or 'infiltrate'" (Sontag 1978:66). A belief in the necessity of war itself, which was shared by certain generations of Americans, has helped to solidify this metaphor: "For the generation of surgeons (and patients) reared during World War II, few questions existed about the necessity for battle—against invading countries or disease. The cause was just, the methods essential, the warrior celebrated" (Cassel 1991:185).

The most dramatic instance of this genre occurs when the disease/enemy is lethal and medicine is expected to defend the body against the formidable foe of death itself. This is, in fact, the very definition of "heroic medicine." Death, conceived of as "defeat," is "one of the basic tenets of the 'technocratic model' that undergirds modern medicine" (Davis-Floyd and St. John 1998:16). Heroic warrior clinicians strategize and mount campaigns against a disease enemy, which has its own tactics and weapons in conquering the body. Cancer serves as a classic example. Treatment here is steeped in military metaphors as patients' bodies are "bombarded" in radiology or "chemically poisoned" in chemotherapy.

Parents with ill children become trained in this language through a host of ways. During one waiting room moment early in her daughter's treatment, Andrena, the mother I introduced at the beginning of this book, read aloud from a pamphlet she had been given on her last visit to the hospital that made explicit the lethal effect of chemotherapy: "This says bone marrow suppression. The drug used to kill cancer cells also kills some normal body cells." She paused to consider this and then remarked steadfastly: "But anyway, I'm gonna find out all about this and then you'll find out too." She declared that she would be "searching for all kinds of information," noting that she had called the hospital, "asking them to send me literature." Andrena once remarked about her daughter's radiation treatments, which were having devastating side effects: "They put the radiation on full blast." She was not simply drawing on common imagery or picking up the informal lingo of the clinic. This trope of the battle also signaled the losses one could expect in any war when one is routinely "blasted"—including, in this case, her child's reduced hearing, balance, and cognitive function.

This genre does not merely assign the body a passive character, however. The body is not merely an unwitting and helpless recipient of hostile invaders. It is also an agent; it too is the site of a complex defense system that can mobilize its own armies to resist invasion through counterattacks. The body comes to be imagined as an internal battleground, as illustrated in Emily Martin's (1994) fascinating account of the ways in which this basic metaphor has taken on particular shadings in different historical periods. For example, Martin describes a shift in American popular culture in the 1960s and 1970s as the body's immune system was reimagined, emerging as an interior defense system that could withstand assaults from deadly invaders who might find their way through the skin's "outer fortifications." By the 1980s, these metaphors were again reconfigured as the immune system became envisioned as a "defended nation state" (1994:54).

Children as well as parents become trained in learning to see their bodies as the site of an internal battle. They may not precisely be the main characters in the canonical version of this genre, but in the battle with chronic illness they too play a role. They are recruited by clinicians to serve as minor characters, assistants in the war. We can see this in the following example. Dr. Johnson, a hematologist, speaks with some enthusiasm about how he made a "little blood model" to facilitate his explanation of being HIV positive or having AIDS. He uses this model especially when he has to disclose to children that they have HIV, and he notes that it is very effective: "Very visual, and the kids, most of the parents, are like, 'Wow.'" His concern is not merely to deliver bad news but to try to ensure compliance in the lifelong regime of taking essential medications.

In the following exchange, Dr. Johnson has decided that it is time to explain to Kenny, who is nine, about his positive HIV status. When Kenny and his grandmother (who is raising him) arrive at his office, he sends Kenny to a play area in the waiting room so that he can talk to his grandmother. He announces that today he wants to tell Kenny about the "germ" in his body. She agrees. When Kenny is called back into Dr. Johnson's office, he brings out his model of white and red blood cells. He tells Kenny that a germ in his body has attacked his white blood cells. He explains that Kenny's white blood cells and T cells got too low and that the medications he has been taking could prevent him from getting sick. Using his model (which looks rather like a "Pac Man" game piece), he illustrates. He places a jack in its "mouth" and the model lights up. The doctor then explains: "HIV is the germ [Pac Man] that attacks and eats white blood cells [the jack] in the body. But the medicine fights the germ." When he is done explaining, Kenny has a few questions.

Kenny: Is what I have worse than sugar diabetes?

Dr. Johnson: Yes.

Kenny: Can friends catch my germ?

Dr. Johnson: Some people are pretty dumb about HIV. They respond like it's a kind of leprosy. But am I nervous about examining you? *(Kenny shakes his head no)* You can't go talking to everyone about what you have. Medicine is so important to keep your T cells fighting strong. Which cell does HIV attack?

Kenny: T cell.

Dr. Johnson: Do you have any other concerns?

Kenny: I'm stuck on the dying part.

Dr. Johnson: You have more chance of dying if you run out into the street and get hit by a truck. You can't die if you don't get sick first. You won't get sick if you take your medicine.

The doctor's words reinforce the message that Kenny's body will mobilize to defend itself if Kenny does his part by faithfully taking his medicine. The doctor may be the general and the strategist of the battle, but the body is expected to cooperate in rallying aid in its own defense, and patient compliance is also necessary to "attack" the "germs" that are destroying the body. When treatment fails and the enemy grows stronger, patients may subtly be blamed or may even blame themselves. What is happening here is not so much that the battle metaphor with its passive patient is abandoned but that the patient himself is reconceived as having his own heroic or at least compliant qualities and responsibilities that can be mobilized to help win the battle against the invading pathogens.[20]

From a family's perspective, the canonical image of biomedicine battling disease takes on further complexity. As in the "detective genre" they may believe they must fight to keep clinicians in the battle. Parents may even come to see themselves, rather than the doctors, as the primary frontline fighters in the battle against disease or death. The following interesting example reveals this as a mother, Noreen, describes herself as having had to become a "Rambo" in caring for her severely ill daughter Danielle, who has sickle-cell anemia. A nurse who has heard Noreen speak to other parents about her experiences caring for her child with sickle-cell disease is vividly struck by Noreen's description of herself as "Rambo mom."

> We did a big parent day on sickle cell. There were over a hundred people who came. And so Mom [Noreen] was one of the speakers. And it was interesting because they were talking about her being a parent of a child with sickle cell, and she said, you know, "What I do is I get in my Rambo mode." She had said, "If my daughter gets just the sniffles, I get hyperalert. I grab all my machine guns, all my equipment, guns there to attack that organism or that whatever. I check the pulse, I listen, you know, watch her color. I do this. I do that." So it's such hyperintense, very vigilant and very, she wants to call everybody, do everything perfect because she's probably scared to death something bad will happen. She's had so many [scares]. [*Her daughter has often become suddenly critically ill and needed to be rushed to the emergency room.*] She said, "I'm the Rambo mom. Gotta get out there and just attack if something happens or just really get things in place."

Like a ferocious warrior, Noreen represents herself as on the front lines of the battlefield, constantly alert to enemy advances in her daughter's body. Fascinatingly, one of the physicians who treats her daughter provides a contrasting description of Noreen. He, too, draws upon the metaphor of battle, but in his account she occupies a considerably diminished position in the "war" they are carrying out. He describes her as a "soldier" in the "trenches." He says, "I mean, I see her kind of, you know, in the trenches, slogging away to try and put away one obstacle at a time."

The rise of new biomedical procedures and life-sustaining technologies offers patients and clinicians new hopes that yet again recast the traditional picture of a battle between a clinician and a disease. Science and technology themselves become the heroic figures in a battle narrative.[21] This recasting also creates new border work for parents. They may take the lead in trying to engage clinicians in experimenting with new strategies of care. Through Internet research and the development of virtual communities formed by people who share a disease, parents discover plentiful information that they then try to bring back to their clinicians. They may attempt to forge alliances with an array of clinicians or clinical sites that they believe are the frontrunners in the battle, those who have new technologies that may advance the war.

For example, Noreen (the "Rambo mom") describes her attempts to get her primary hematologist to investigate some experimental research she has read about on a sickle-cell Web site. As part of this effort, she takes a trip to another research hospital where, in her view, "they're more aggressive with their research" than the hospital where her daughter is currently treated. She believes that if she does this investigation perhaps she can motivate her hematologist to take a more aggressive stance in getting her own daughter into experimental research projects. She offers the following hypothetical conversation she plans on having with her doctor when she brings back this new information:

> Look, Doctor, this is what they are doing over there, here it is. Why don't you give them a call and you speak with them and see what they are doing? And see if this is something that you might be interested in.

This imagined conversation is based upon past experiences where she has tried to bring new information to the clinicians treating her daughter. She sees this as one of the roles she has come to play.

> You know, I think they [the treating clinicians] started calling me their eyes and ears. They said, "Oh, she knows. Send her [to conferences, etc.] because she always reports back."

She reinforces her frontline role, recounting a recent conversation with a hematologist at another clinical center who tells her about the research they have been doing on sickle cell disease and its relationship to pulmonary disease (which her daughter also suffers from). She describes their conversation with enthusiasm. "We've got our sickle mouse and our sickle rat," he tells her, "and we're working with pulmonary doctors." She concludes:

> He gives me a rundown of what they're doing. And I'm like, "Great! Which one of these things can my daughter participate in?"

Healing as Machine Repair

A third canonical genre portrays the body as machine, a biomechanical metaphor offering one of the "basic tenets of the 'technocratic model' that undergirds modern medicine" (Davis-Floyd and St. John 1998:16), in which "nature, society and the human body came to be viewed as an assemblage of interchangeable parts that could be repaired or replaced from the outside" (Davis-Floyd and St. John 1998:19). As a machine, the body is potentially "fixable": "The implicit genesis of illness is an unlucky breakdown in a body that is conceived on mechanistic lines" (A. Frank 1995:88). This machine metaphor is not at all abstract, some mere philosophical conceit. It belongs to medical common sense, as an implicit part of our cultural narrative of illness and healing, and is routinely taken quite literally.[22] In canonical terms, the clinician operates as a kind of supertechnician, a supermechanic. The drama of this genre is especially apparent in certain clinical practices like surgical and rehabilitation specialties or with certain illnesses like heart disease.

This genre not only is called upon by clinicians to describe their work, but, like the other canonical genres, has been incorporated into popular cultural perceptions of the body, especially the heart. In Weiss's (1997) terms, the "heart attack body is a machine." Martin (1994) has called it a "Fordist body," a kind of assembly-line body. This picture of the body has been aided by dramatic and comparatively recent surgical interventions, especially the possibility of replacing ailing body parts with "new ones" that are either mechanical or donated organs. Of the three genres, that of the body as machine can confer on the surgeon the most heroic and mythical qualities, for he plies a terrifyingly risky trade in which, with knife in hand, he aggressively slices into the body in order to heal it (Cassel 1991).

Families learn to speak in a language of bodies and their parts, as when a grandmother, Summer, describes her grandchild's surgery for his congenital foot deformities. She offers the matter-of-fact language of mechanical repair, describing the body parts that the surgeons "made," "straightened," and "turned around." As she portrays these procedures, she conveys an image of her grandson being transformed, quite literally, into a kind of machine, a body held together with "bolts":

> When he was born both feet was flat. . . . He had no ankle. They had to do a pinky toe. They had to make a toe. And they also had to make an ankle and then they had to straighten, they had to break his feet. Break them and then straighten him out. Turn them around. Turn them all around. So they put the bolts and stuff in.

Parents faced with ongoing medical issues with their child often express a longing to have doctors who can "just fix things," even if these are not the most crucial problems for their child's health. A mother reports how much she liked a surgeon her daughter saw because although he was called in "to do something else, he's like, 'Oh by the way, I'll fix this for you.'" He was referring to a hernia her daughter had (in addition to more serious problems), and the mother repeats his easy assurance about the hernia repair, "We can fix that." "So it was nice," she concludes. Here, the ability to fix something in her daughter's body, however comparatively minor, becomes a hopeful sign that the body is, indeed, sometimes and in some respects, actually fixable.

The institutional structure of health care with its array of specialists helps to keep a narrow focus on biomedical practice as directed to repairing isolated body parts. For example, rehabilitation therapists often do not have any direct contact with physicians who are treating the same children. They may not even be aware of the actual diagnosis, but they do not necessarily see this as an impediment to treatment. After all, they are supposed to work only on fixing a finite set of body problems. A rehabilitation therapist says that while it might be good to know the diagnosis and the disease process in detail, it is often not necessary because body repair of isolated nonfunction is really the point of her job: "It doesn't really matter that much except in terms of how is it going to progress. I mean you are really looking at what is wrong. And how can you fix it. And what can you do to improve it." Clinicians often complain that parents erroneously assume that they can simply fix what is wrong with their chronically ill child. A surgeon comments:

> The biggest risk for any surgeon is unrealistic expectations. People have an idea that they have an operation and then they'll be perfect again. And my

idea of a good expectation or a good outcome and their idea of a good outcome may be totally different. So that it's important during the description of the operation to make sure that they have a good idea of what a good outcome is. Second is to actually focus them on that idea of expectations between them and me may be different.

Sometimes a family's "false hopes" or "unrealistic expectations" place them in the category of problem parents from the clinician's perspective. A doctor reports the following typical conversation with "some selected families."

> There are selected families where they bring in the kid and they say, "You fix them." Period. "Well, you need to follow up." "No, I don't wanna do that. You call the therapist for me." So, there are families that don't do what they should be doing as parents.

An occupational therapist echoes this complaint but also sees it as her job to "educate the parent."

> I tend to start therapy when I first introduce myself to the parent. I tell them what OT [occupational therapy] is all about, what our goals are. I pretty much start off the conversation with "You realize that one hour a week is not going to do anything." And I think that some of them are surprised by it, because they think that they are going to come and get fixed. And it does seem to help a lot. Changing their—the way they see therapy. It is not a cure-all. It is a teaching tool. Because I think that some parents think that, "This is great. It's a break. I'm going to go down and get coffee." You know, sometimes that is fine. I'll let them do that, but they have to spend the last fifteen minutes with me and review what I have done.

While clinicians often believe that parents have unrealistic expectations about what kind of fixing can be expected, unsurprisingly parents offer a different picture. Many admit that when they first received a diagnosis, even of a chronic illness, they could not help but hope that their child could just be "fixed," like a car that had been dropped off at the garage. But this picture changes over time as they gradually come to realize what they are facing and what their child's possibilities are. A mother describes her own shifting understanding of her child's sickle-cell disease and the slow movement from hoping that her daughter could just be "fixed" to a recognition that fixing was not an option—that this was going to be a lifetime medical problem. She describes her initial attitude when her child was born premature and in the neonatal intensive care unit (NICU):

> Yeah, I wanted to fix the disease. Most parents, I think when your kids are sick, you know how we are, we want to fix them. "I don't care what you

do," you tell the doctor. "Just fix them so I can take my kid home." When she was in the NICU, they said to me, "We're going to put her in an incubator, we're going to grow her, we're going to fix this, then you can take your baby home!" So, I figure whatever they were doing was working. She's growing. She's developing. She doesn't have any hemorrhages that they told me about. Um, yeah, she has some lung problems, but we caught—we're dealing with those. We're treating the problem. She'll outgrow all of this!

As the years have passed, she has come to appreciate that her primary doctor does not promise that he can simply "fix" her child, for she realizes that this is no longer an option. At least she gets an honest doctor, one whom she can trust.

> One thing I like about this doctor is he never says he can fix it, but he tries. He's the old professor and kinda like a father figure, I suppose, in a sense . . . and I'm just so appreciative that he agreed to take us on as his patients in the first place from the very day that he looked at my daughter's X-rays. He looked at her medical records, her history, and he looked at all of that and he said, "I'll take her." And it's been great. It's been a great relationship with him ever since. And it's nice because my initial desire was to just find a doctor that would fix the problem and make it go away. And now that I'm realizing that there is not only, it is not something that's gonna go away anytime soon.

This mother illustrates how hope can shift from a narrowly defined idea of fixing a broken body to an idea of developing a partnership with a clinician who will tell you what can and cannot be fixed. But this chronic illness is also very hard for her, her child, and her family. It is this relationship and her trust in the doctor and other clinicians on the sickle-cell team that bring with it, as she says, "little rays of hope [because] these people actually care."

In the following exchange, a surgeon, Dr. Sanderson, draws upon the imagery of body as broken machine to try to impress upon the parents (Andrew and Darlene) of a critically ill child (Arlene) that the infant should be taken off life support. They do not agree. This exchange is part of an ongoing battle between the clinical staff and the parents. In fact, their resistance to taking their child off life support caused enormous disturbance and disagreements among the clinicians caring for Arlene. One can hear almost a kind of desperation in Dr. Sanderson's relentless cataloguing of body breakdowns "from head to toe" and how deeply machine imagery is embedded in the clinical imaginary. It is almost as though he is telling the parents that their daughter has become too much of a machine, that the failure of her internal machinery in so many critical functions and her reliance on these external machines mean she is, in effect, dead.

As the parents stand together in the NICU next to their daughter's bed, a social worker also by their side, the doctor begins:

> *Dr. Sanderson:* I want to start by describing her conditions from head to toe. I have spent quite a bit of time with her and have seen her progress. I want to start with her lungs. She no longer breathes by herself. Several times during the day, we have to bag her for long periods of time just to bring her back from death. Sometimes the ventilator is not enough because her body is making so many secretions they are blocking the lungs and airways. Her stents, which have been replaced several times, are collapsing down and might be clogging her lungs. . . . In order to just get rid of the secretions, we have to detach her from the machine, which makes her desaturate. Her vent settings are almost at their maximum, and for someone her size so much pressure damages the lungs more and more. Her lungs are getting worse and worse, and it's harder and harder to keep her alive. *(Dr. Sanderson is then interrupted by the social worker, who is also present. He quickly answers her question and returns to his catalog.)* Another thing is her heart. Her heart is beating slower and slower. Because of her heart disease, it needs to work harder to pump blood through her body. When the lungs are bad, it's harder and harder on her heart. We could try to fix the heart, but she wouldn't survive the surgery. So to fix her heart is not an option. You have that going downhill too. Next is her feeding. She is not able to eat through her G-tube anymore.

> *Darlene:* Why?

> *Dr. Sanderson:* Because her breathing is so bad, it's not safe to give her food that might come back up. She is now getting all her nutrition through an IV.

> *Darlene:* As long as she gets nutrition.

> *Dr. Sanderson: (jumps in quickly)* So she's able to get nutrition intravenously, but the longer she's on TPN [total parenteral nutrition] the harder it is to go back to food. The last thing, then, is she used to open her eyes a lot more. In the last month in my opinion she's more and more uncomfortable and having a harder and harder time breathing. All these interventions of bagging her and pounding her chest are taking a toll on her. She is less and less responsive. She's not responding. Neurologically she did not have a lot to start with. She just barely has enough to keep her heart going. Just enough to get by.

Having presented this long list of critical problems with the child, the doctor sums up, offering his conclusion (phrased as a question) that in the face of such massive machine breakdown, keeping her on life support is not the "best thing for this child":

Dr. Sanderson: What I ask myself every time I walk into her room is, "Am I doing the best thing for this child?" That's the question I ask myself.

Andrew: Yes. Yes. We don't want to take her off the machines. When she goes, she's going to go on her own. That's how I believe. That's how she'll fight it out.

Dr. Sanderson: As long as you know that it's not her but the machines that are keeping her alive.

Andrew: The only thing stopping her from dying is the machines and medicine. We understand that.

This final exchange is interesting on both sides. From the clinical perspective, one sees how the machine image offers a potent organizing plot structure—a narrative of the impossibility of keeping any part fixed for long. As soon as one thing is even temporarily repaired, something else begins to break down, or the very fixing causes damage to another part. And, that engine of the machine metaphor—the heart—can barely be kept going. But if Dr. Sanderson's conclusion is that she should be pulled off life support because at this stage nothing more than the external machines that are "keeping her alive," he also invokes the limit of this trope. His words also convey something else, even something contradictory. Unlike a machine (which presumably feels nothing), this is a living child who is being subjected to the painful, horrific interventions needed, "bagging" and "pounding," as she continually hovers near death. He tries to impress upon the parents the cruelty of this procedure, the pain it is causing their daughter.

If the physician's words have a complexity that complicates the canonical, Andrew's response is even subtler and, from the clinician's perspective, baffling. Although he appears to agree with the doctor, assuring him that he and Darlene "understand that the only thing stopping her from dying is the machines and the medicine," he does not agree with Dr. Sanderson's conclusions. Why is this? To get a better sense of these parents' perspective, I need to introduce the fourth healing genre.

"I'm Stuck on the Dying Part" and Other Troubles: Healing as Transformative Journey

Sometimes healing is conceived as a transformative journey. This is the central genre invoked by the families and, as children get older, by them as well. Personal and often social transformation is at the heart of this narrative genre; broadly speaking, it concerns what Arthur Frank (1995) calls a "quest."[23] This is not a journey that families (or patients) want to undertake but one they are plunged into, thanks to the illness or disability they face. This is also the quintessential border genre. In this dramatic genre, the patient and family, rather than the clinicians, emerge as key protagonists. It is not that canonical plots are unimportant from the parents' perspective; rather, they are imagined as subplots within narrative frames that encompass personal, familial, and community lives. Families frequently express a concern to find clinicians who will *also* embrace and accompany them on a journey where hopes may change, where they may even have to encompass the death of a child.

This genre is impossible to speak about without invoking the eventful and especially the personal side of illness. The idea that one lives a life—which is, in some way, one's own and which is even a moral project—is an indispensable feature of this genre. The phenomenon of bodily affliction changes too, becoming situated within a social web of any number of other afflictions and quandaries—existential, practical, political, economic, ethical—that engage patients, the families, and at times the clinicians as well.

When nine-year-old Kenny hears from his physician that he is HIV positive and remarks, when asked if he has any questions, that he is "stuck on the dying part," the hematologist answers confidently: "You have more chance of getting hit by a bus" if medications are taken as prescribed. This answer, though perfectly fitting the canonical plot of battling disease, elides another drama that underlies Kenny's question, one that arises out of his personal and family history. What kind of story am I in? he is asking. He has a mother he rarely sees but knows is often quite ill. (She has AIDS.) His initial question to Dr. Johnson, "Is what I have worse than sugar diabetes," is also not an abstract clinical question but an intimately personal one. His grandparents are raising him. They are his primary family. At the time of this session his grandfather was a very seriously ill diabetic who, thanks to the diabetes, had already had a foot amputated. He was, in fact, dying. So when Dr. Johnson quickly tells Kenny that what he has is, in fact, worse than "sugar diabetes," he is missing the kind of question Kenny is asking.

The practice of hope families are engaged in is often deeply connected to notions of personal transformation and to the idea of life as a kind of journey that demands self-transformation. Hope, in this genre, can in no way be reduced to "success" or "cure" in any simple sense. Science, biotechnology, and clinical experts are no longer primary protagonists, though they still have their parts to play. If it were not for the pervasiveness, indeed the centrality, of this genre among the families in this study, I might have chosen simply to write about "clinical hope" or "biomedical hope." But, as I argued at the outset, the sort of hope that biomedicine and biotechnology can provide (or serve to promise at some future time) is only a small part of the picture of hope from the perspective of these families. Hope cannot be reduced to this canonical portrait. Instead, this is the genre of "blues hope."

It is remarkable how often patients or their families portray hope as a journey that requires not merely a transformation of the body but the transformation of a person's, a family's, or even a community's whole life. When Sandra finally finds out that her four-month-old infant has cerebral palsy, thanks to Sandra's mother, who confronts her physician and gets him to refer the infant to a specialist, this is not merely a clinical matter. Sandra tells her story as part of a narrative of how she had to transform herself to become a good mother to her severely disabled child. She had to learn to fight, to become (to use Noreen's terminology) a "Rambo mom." She had to "find strength," not just to bear the difficulties of raising a medically fragile child, but also to learn how to battle physicians when necessary. Hope depends, in large part, on such efforts of transformation.

One of the enduring themes of this dramatic genre is the way illness remakes the social world for the sufferer: "transforming the society of the patient by constriction, recasting, concentration, and consolidation" (Hahn 1985:92). We encounter this theme in a particularly vivid way in the plethora of memoirs patients have written about their experience of illness and healing. In addition to the impoverishment of life, which one might expect, there is often a surprising sense in which—as Paul Stoller remarks of his own experience of cancer—one may "incorporate illness" into one's being, perpetuating "a deeper understanding of life's forces and meanings" (2004:202–3). This insistence on incorporating an illness into personal and family life is voiced again and again by the families in this research and constitutes one of the most important themes of this book.[24]

It might seem that this narrative genre would be completely outside or even antagonistic to clinical medicine. And, in fact, it was rarely made explicit by most of the clinicians in our study. However, there were exceptions, and this genre is also garnering some attention in the clinical community more broadly. The idea that serious illness involves a kind of biographical breakdown (a "lesion in the self," as Oliver Sacks [1984:67] has said), that it must be understood biographically and through the use of narrative, is not new to some specialties of biomedicine, especially psychiatry.[25] In recent years this narrative genre of the journey has also gained visibility in the clinical world, in physical medicine, as an aspect of a movement that has arisen among clinicians themselves, variously entitled "narrative medicine" (Charon 2006) and "narrative-based medicine" (Hurwitz, Greenhalgh, and Skultans 2004).[26]

It is not surprising that a dramatic genre that invokes healing as an *experience* should call upon "the journey" as a central image. Etymologically, the term *experience* in Western languages has been associated not only with a kind of journey but with one that involves both perils and experiences from which one learns. "Insofar as 'to try' *(expereri)* contains the same root as *periculum,* or 'danger,' there is also a covert association between experience and peril, which suggests that it comes from having survived risks and learned something from the encounter (*ex* meaning a coming forth from)" (Jay 2005:10). This philosophical consideration has close ties to a much older religious tradition: experience as religious journey. The quite specific religious associations with the notion of experience also have a significant history in Western culture (Jay 2005; Taylor 1989, 2007).

But the spiritual resonance of autobiographical accounts of illness that are prevalent in the literature even by those who are not "religious" is especially intriguing. The "journey" is often depicted as having the kind of liminality that we associate with, for example, Victor Turner's (1969) rituals of transformation. The hospital itself becomes a liminal site, an "in-between" space. Patients—as Sacks in his autobiographical account of recovery from a severe leg injury puts it—are, by virtue of their illnesses, forced to descend "to great darknesses and depths" and then "like pilgrims" must try to find their way out of "the sheer misery, the storms and terrors, of sickness" (Sacks 1984:145).

Parents often explicitly call upon the religious connotations of this genre. I return now to the exchange between Dr. Sanderson and the parents of Arlene, the critically ill infant on life support. Why do the parents agree with the physician that their child would die without these external machines, that every system is faltering or failing, and that she has been on the brink of death many times, yet disagree with his conclusion? Why do they speak of their child as "having a fighting spirit," as they do in this exchange and as they very often insisted in interviews? (They also told many of their own stories about these harrowing back-from-death moments in the eighteen months their daughter lived.) They are intensely religious people. For them, this genre of transformative journey spans much more than a human life. It speaks to a much grander history. The practice of medicine and its machinery are just a short story in a cosmological narrative. From their perspective, the clinicians simply misunderstand their own role in human history. They seem to believe that they (or these parents) should be in charge of life and death. But this is not a human matter. It is about hoping, struggling to hope, doing everything possible to sustain life while at the same time recognizing that life and death are not fully under human control. For them, the practice of healing (and the hope of healing) invokes a plot that brings in an array of cosmological actors. Not only does this narrative encompass the personal, the interpersonal, and the structural—it is on a scale such that all of human history and its creations constitute one small episode in a much vaster epic.

If hope is a border drama, its borders encompass horizons that extend far beyond the activities and actors of the clinical setting. It is this sense that clinical plots are necessarily little tales, moments (however eventful) in other histories, that families hope clinicians will recognize. Not all the families I will write about are religious in the manner of Andrew and Darlene. However, the sense of hope and healing as tied to pilgrimage is deeply embedded in their way of understanding the situations they face and the kind of story they struggle to carry out. More than any of the other genres, this one speaks to the potential tragedy that haunts hope, for there is no obvious ending to this journey, and, in any case, moral pilgrims may not be able to endure its travails.

CHAPTER 3

Border Trouble

Thus far, I have outlined (with increasing ethnographic illustration) a narrative phenomenology of practice. Although I have given a number of concrete examples to support my assertions, arguments, and taxonomies, a good deal of this discussion has been in the abstract. This chapter marks a shift to extended examinations of particular people, places, and events, centering upon the primary families that provide the focal point for this book. I open this ethnographic scene not with them or with any hospitals or clinics, however. Taking a step back, I begin with a brief historical and demographic portrait of the contexts that have been so influential in shaping clinical care for African Americans in Los Angeles.

LOS ANGELES AS A CULTURAL BORDER ZONE: THE AFRICAN AMERICAN EXPERIENCE

For someone familiar with poor urban communities in America's northern cities, Los Angeles is anomalous. Having worked and lived in underclass black and Irish neighborhoods in Chicago and Boston, I was very unprepared for it. In Boston and Chicago, when you are in a poor area you know it. But when I first moved to Los Angeles it all seemed so much more suburban. Some of the most impoverished families in our study lived in houses with tree-lined streets and neatly groomed lawns. Even when front yards were more packed dirt than grass, one might see a surprising burst of bougainvillea climbing cheerily up a wall or running along a fence. In the spring, you could smell the jasmine. I was accustomed to a grittier look: tightly packed, rundown apartment buildings with boarded-up windows. Instead of this barren landscape, there were cactus and exotic palms and flowers of a dozen different colors. There were places to park just as you might find in any suburb. Granted, the commercial streets looked pretty shabby, but even so, poverty had a different face when you drove through many of the neighborhoods.

There was another difference. The poor neighborhoods in the northern cities I knew best were nearly always close to the urban center. What I was seeing in L.A. reflected a demographic pattern that is in some ways unique to the early black settlement of this city. Perhaps the bougainvilleas and the tree-lined streets that surprised me when I arrived in the mid-1990s were vestiges of the early years of African American experience in Los Angeles. African Americans began migrating to Los Angeles as far back as the 1880s, moving west as the railroads were extended and working as porters or waiters on the trains. But the more significant migration happened a few years later, in the early decades of the twentieth century, as African Americans left the rural South in search of work and a better life. Many came from Texas and Louisiana.

While there has historically been a concentration of African Americans in traditional neighborhoods of South Central, Watts, and the near downtown, beginning in the 1950s and 1960s black neighborhoods have also grown up in many other outposts: in a Venice neighborhood by the beach, in Altadena right next to posh, old-money Pasadena, and in pockets of the San Fernando Valley. The central urban black area continued to grow in size and population through the 1960s and 1970s even while those urban/suburban black communities far from the center also continued to develop.

This demographic of African American immigrants from Texas and Louisiana holds generally true for the families in our study, even a hundred years after the earliest migrants. Although there is certainly a geographic spread among them (a few families come from New York, two have Belizean ancestry, and one is from Nigeria), most trace their roots to these areas of the rural South. Many still have ties to extended family "back home," and some express a nostalgic hope that one day they will be able to leave the city and return to these rural homelands. One of the families did, in fact, move to Texas to live near her relatives, though four years later she is still uncertain whether this was a good decision. She often contemplates a return to L.A. Life in the South inevitably brings its problems too. Some families have told graphic stories about their own experiences of violence in the southern states where they grew up that precipitated their relocation to Los Angeles. One grandmother, Cadence, now in her midsixties, told this story about how she had been sent to L.A. by her mother in the mid-1950s after having spent her early childhood in Texas.

> I remember, I remember I was, I don't remember how old I was, but I remember Emmett Till, when he was killed. Emmett Till was a boy, in the South. And they say he had gone, he was in, I don't know what southern town, visiting some relatives. He was, he had come from Chicago or somewhere. Anyway, the story goes that he whistled at a white woman. And he was crucified. He—they—they tortured him and—and killed him, and mutilated his body. And I always remember as a child, I never will forget it, when that happened, my mother made a decision, that she is gonna send us from Texas (that was in the height of the civil rights movement), she was gonna send us from Texas to California. Yeah, 'cause we never had any problems, other than, you know, . . . we knew, about racism. But when they killed him, he was fourteen years old. . . . Yeah, fourteen years old, and they hung him. They threw him in the river. They did a little bit of everything. They mutilated him so badly that his mother didn't even recognize him. And I remember looking into, at that time, this black magazine, *Jet* magazine, and seeing the picture of this boy. And it scared me to death. And it scared my mother too. And so she made a decision. She says, "I'm gonna send you guys to California," to my mother's sister, who was here, in California. And she sent us out here in the fifties.

Los Angeles was far from a racial utopia during that time, but it stood as a beacon of hope and comparative safety when contrasted with the images of white southern violence that were so vividly apparent during the civil rights era.

There is a certain "Paradise lost" quality to the African American historical experience in Los Angeles. At the turn of the twentieth century several features of Los Angeles were especially appealing to blacks considering a move out west, including a sense of less blatant racism compared to the northern cities, greater possibilities of home ownership, and greater job opportunities. In addition, there was the good weather, clean air scented with orange blossoms (or so it was advertised to the rest of the country), and a "sunshine city" optimism that propelled black migrants from the South just as it lured whites from the states of the northern Midwest. As Lonnie Bunche puts it: "California's call of hope and opportunity has had a powerful effect on Afro-Americans, a people who, at times, have had little more than faith, hope and dreams to sustain themselves" (1990:102).

The first thirty years of the twentieth century marked what has been called the "Golden Era" for African Americans in Los Angeles. This was an era characterized by a growing, community-spirited black population, the rise of black church and civic associations that supported black businesses and education, a lively developing cultural, artistic, and night life along Central Street, and relative harmony with other ethnic and racial groups. These were decades remembered nostalgically by mid- and late-century African Americans who saw the post–World War II decades bring increasing social, economic, and political problems and a loss of the community solidarity that had characterized much of the century's first half.

During those early decades of the twentieth century, blacks viewed Los Angeles as a "kind of racial paradise for African Americans" (Sides 2004:11). For example, W. E. B. Du Bois wrote in 1913, just after visiting the city: "Los Angeles was wonderful. The air was scented with orange blossoms and the beautiful homes lay low crouching on the earth as though they loved its scents and flowers. Nowhere in the United States is the Negro so well and beautifully housed, nor the average efficiency and intelligence in the colored population so high. Here is an aggressive, hopeful group—with some wealth, large industrial opportunity and a buoyant spirit."

One of the city's biggest attractions was home ownership. It was easier for African Americans to purchase homes in Los Angeles than in any northern city, as exemplified by these startling statistics: "In 1910, almost 40 percent of African Americans in Los Angeles County owned their homes, as compared to only 2.4 percent in New York and 8 percent in Chicago" (Sides 2004:15). The fact that the black community was always comparatively small (ranging from about 3 percent in the beginning to a high of about 18 percent in 1970) may have helped in the early years to make home ownership laws less restrictive and to mitigate against the apartheid-like settlement patterns one immediately notices in cities like Chicago, Detroit, or Cleveland. However, the main thing that has historically made home ownership more possible in Los Angeles than other cities (until recent decades) is the sheer vast size of the city itself and its relatively low population density. This kept housing prices comparatively low for a very long time.

In addition to the possibility of buying a home, California as a whole has historically had less restrictive racial segregation laws for schools and employment. Los Angeles, in particular, was highly multiethnic from the start, and in the early decades Mexican and Japanese Americans lived in close proximity to African Americans. There was a sense among blacks that race and ethnicity did not matter as much as they did in other cities. Or perhaps it was just that prejudice could be directed to a broader range of ethnic groups and people of color than in most other American cities. An essay published in 1911 in the black newspaper *The Liberator* put it succinctly and ironically: "Perhaps the presence in this section of the country in large numbers of the representatives of every nation on the globe, has much to do with the success that has attended our men, as representatives of the so called 'backward races'; they have no monopoly of the embarrassing attention and prejudice so often directed mainly at them" (quoted in Bunche 1990:104).

Immense ethnic diversity in a comparatively compact area of Central and South Central Los Angeles also occurred during these settlement decades because of the effect of covenants established early in the century to protect white (and mostly Protestant) neighborhoods from all nonwhite groups, including initially Italians. Asian immigrants, Mexicans, and Italians moved into the same downtown and South Central neighborhoods that blacks occupied as they were denied housing access in these "whites only" zones. Despite some ethnic diversity, a strong, geographically centralized African American community was able to fight the city government collectively for rights, especially the right to integration. Property ownership rights, the right to equal labor, and basic social rights were gradually won. Increasingly, African Americans had the legal possibility of moving into areas that had once been restricted to whites.

During World War II, new waves of African American immigrants poured into the city as employment opportunities opened up. Los Angeles had a great deal of war-related industry that provided well-paid work. While blacks had been excluded from this lucrative sector, they were finally able to win the right to employment in it. (Roosevelt himself was forced to step in under pressure from black activists across the country.) This offered new prosperity for African Americans. Unfortunately, increasingly restrictive housing regulations meant that they became more and more crowded into the South Central area of the city.

Since this mid-twentieth-century boom period, two important events have contributed to the downfall of the Los Angeleno "American Dream" that once drew blacks to the city. The most important has been the continued decline of blue-collar manufacturing throughout the country that has wreaked havoc on all black urban communities. For Los Angeles, this has meant the closing of major automobile and tire factories, shipyards, and steel plants. In tandem with the loss of these economic opportunities has been the notorious rise of drug and gang activity.

These devastating realities, coupled with the lessening of housing segregation laws, meant that by 1980 the residential pattern for blacks in Los Angeles began to change in earnest. There was increasing out-migration. The South Central area (including Watts and Compton) started shrinking as more blacks moved to outlying areas in Los Angeles County. Middle-class African Americans moved to safer and more prestigious areas of the city, removing the base of financial and political support that had been part of the original African American experience in Los Angeles. The immensely wide gap between rich and poor, characteristic of Los Angeles as a whole, has affected the African American community by splitting it increasingly into disparate social classes.

At the beginning of the twenty-first century, this out-migration had yet another face. It represented a movement of even the very poor to distant suburban communities where there was more affordable housing and the hope of increased safety. More recently, new black communities have also emerged in far-flung high desert suburbs, two hours' drive from the central city. Many of the families in our study have moved several times since we began, often out of central city neighborhoods and into these more distant communities. The Rodney King race riots of 1994 propelled many families to move to areas they perceived as less violent and safer for their children. The reduction in the supply of government-subsidized housing has contributed to this shifting demographic.

The pressure of a fast-growing Latino community may also be influencing this out-migration from the urban center. In recent decades, Mexican Americans and other Central American ethnic groups, as well as Asian Americans, have been rapidly expanding from East Los Angeles (where they were once primarily concentrated) into the South Central area, a pattern that continues to this day. This expansion has brought rising tension between these various groups, particularly Latinos and blacks, as they compete over housing, jobs, and political and economic resources.

This tension is reflected in clinical settings. Urban hospitals in Los Angeles reveal a multicultural face that is often far from peaceful. The unfortunate recent history of the Martin Luther King–Drew Medical Center provides a vivid example. One of the results of the Watts riots in the mid-1960s was that the city agreed to found a hospital in the area that would serve the local community. Since its opening it has been a black-run hospital. Though sorely needed (there were no hospitals in the area before it was built) and a source of tremendous pride among African Americans, it has also been a site of immense controversy and conflict. It has been systematically underfunded over the years, has operated on a financial shoestring, and has been threatened frequently with budget cuts by the city. This hospital has not been a major clinical site for the families in our study, even for those who live near it. While some have expressed pride in having a predominantly black-run hospital in Los Angeles, several have also been concerned about the quality of care available. (It acquired the unhappy local nickname "Killer King.")

In recent years, as the demographics of the South Central area have changed, there has been pressure by other ethnic groups, particularly the Latino community, to shift the hospital's administrative power away from blacks. An excerpt from a newspaper article sums it up:

> Most of the patients and visitors in the hospital are Latino, not black. Many are holding conversations in Spanish. And increasingly, they are pressing the hospital to hire doctors and other top staff members who look and talk like them—a demand Latino leaders say is met largely with indifference, if not indignation, from the hospital's black managers and its political patrons. . . .
>
> The change rumbling through King hospital is just a fraction of the fallout from a seismic shift in the racial makeup of Los Angeles County. In 1960, four out of five people in the county were white. But a wave of immigration has transformed the jurisdiction into one where no ethnic or racial group holds the majority. The county's population of 9.5 million is now 41 percent Hispanic, 37 percent white, 11 percent Asian and 10 percent black. The Latino and Asian population each have more than doubled in the past 20 years, dramatically alternating the dynamics of race here. (Fletcher 1998:A1)

In the summer of 2008, amid immense local controversy, the hospital was essentially shut down by the city, leaving, yet again, no emergency room within miles of the Watts and South Central area (Rabbani 2008).

This brief look at African Americans' settlement history in Los Angeles demonstrates how the demographics of contemporary Los Angeles dictate that any major hospital necessarily operates as a cultural border zone, serving, and likely being staffed by, a widely diverse ethnic and racial community. The clashes and the kind of wariness and mistrust one can find in Los Angeles urban hospitals are not, of course, particular to this city. They also reflect a national struggle around race that has marked the African American experience for three centuries.

CLINICAL CARE AS BORDER TRAVEL: RACE AND MEDICINE

City hospitals in a multicultural metropolis like Los Angeles are further characterized by pluralisms of class, race, language, and culture that routinely trip everyone up. Such culturally based confusions and difficulties have become an increasing focus of attention for clinicians and medical anthropologists alike, spawning continued efforts to cultivate the "cultural competence" of health professionals (e.g., Hunt 2004, 2005; Lakes, Lopez, and Garro 2006, though the literature on this is vast). In many hospitals in Los Angeles, you can stand still for five minutes in any one spot, or ride up the elevator from the first to the third floor, and be almost guaranteed to hear at least three different languages: English and Spanish, of course, but also potentially Korean, Mandarin, Cantonese, Vietnamese, Arabic, Tagalog, Japanese, Farsi, Armenian, and dozens more, especially if you count the dialects. I have lived in American cities all my adult life, but the only other time I have seen such breadth of ethnic diversity in as concentrated a space is in certain airports. Heathrow comes to mind, as well as Frankfurt, Delhi, and New York's JFK.

This multiculturalism is by no means unique to hospitals in Los Angeles. At both policy and personal levels, the problem of border crossing is intensifying in health care. Massive migrations to the United States have meant that health care, especially in many urban settings, is characterized by a dizzying array of languages, nationalities, racial identifications, social classes, and religions. And this phenomenon is increasing at a rapid pace. The United States is growing more ethnically diverse, and this means that health care increasingly involves providing treatment for diverse populations. Diversity is very often accompanied by unequal access to care. For African Americans in particular, race plays a central role in adverse health outcomes (Porter 1994). Extensive research already exists on this issue, and I will highlight only a few well-documented points that have also emerged as primary for the families in our study. My purpose throughout this book is less to add further documentation to an already impressive body of evidence concerning racial discrimination and health disparities than to explore how perceptions of racial discrimination and subtle discriminatory practices are enacted in clinical encounters and how they influence the practice of hope.

How do the dramatic healing genres and narrative activities I outlined in earlier chapters help shape suspicions, misunderstandings, and discriminatory dramas? Everyday narrative activities such as mind reading, storytelling, and emplotting of action provide primary vehicles through which structural conditions, identities, and power/knowledge discourses are concretely realized. They are realized not as necessary or inevitable workings of macrostructures but as intimate dramas of dismissal, even in the face of grave need. The African American families I speak of here respond by struggling to understand how and why they cannot get care for their children and how they might learn any "cultural competencies" that could help them master their perilous journey through the worlds of health care. In turning to narrative as an analytic frame, then, I am trying to keep alive the uncertainty, suspense, and possibility of everyday social practices. I have in mind not only the kind that points toward the potential for social improvement but also the darker possibilities latent in everyday actions, those that reveal the dangers inherent in what may appear to many participants—especially clinicians—as benign, insignificant, or even beneficent.

African American parents in our study find themselves trying to "read the minds" of health professionals to discern whether they are being discriminated against. As one frustrated father put it about his many trips to the emergency room with his very ill daughter:

> Sometimes you are just going through emergency, you . . . been there two or three, four hours. Then you see Hispanic kids come through or white kids come through. And all of a sudden you notice they done went through. But we still sitting. You know, sometimes that tends to reflect in my head, "What the hell is going on?"

Family members may conduct their own tests to see if their suspicions hold out. A mother once said she had at first been quite sure that she was being made to wait longer because she was black. But then she noted when others were called, and when she saw that several white families were waiting just as long she concluded with relief that she was not being singled out.

When families describe their fears of racial profiling, their worries are reflected in a wealth of research concerning connections between health disparities and race in the United States, particularly for African Americans. Here I will just note a few illustrative studies. African Americans are far more likely than other ethnic racial groups to believe that race is a problem in health care,[1] and, unsurprisingly, there is tremendous evidence that such discrimination does occur.[2] They are persistently a minority group where the most dramatic disparities have been documented, disparities apparent across a broad range of illness categories.[3] They are also routinely subjected to the greatest racial stereotyping and have the least access to health services.[4] Researchers have found that African American patients are likely to be seen by physicians as more "at risk" for noncompliance, more lacking in adequate social support, less educated, and less intelligent than white patients.[5]

I have been speaking of race, but especially when considering the situation of African Americans it is necessary to examine the link between race and class (Wilson 2009). With regard to the hospital as a cultural border zone, the realities of poverty are extremely significant. Most, though not all, of the families I describe in this book are members of the underclass—a class that is growing in numbers as the gap between the rich and the impoverished continues to widen, particularly in Los Angeles. While, as Goldberg notes, "in the public mind of America, 'black' and 'under-class' have tended to become synonymous" (1997:130), the picture is more complex. The current socioeconomic situation for African Americans as a whole is by no means homogeneous. Roughly one-third of African Americans are now middle class. But the numbers of those who fall below the poverty line continue to grow as well.

Health Care in the United States: A Brief Overview

To understand why health disparities are so great for African Americans, especially as compared to whites, it is also useful to place this question within the context of the way that health care is delivered and paid for in the United States. This is a complicated issue, and this book is by no means devoted to the political economy of health care. But a broad sketch may be helpful here.[6] Health care is uniquely structured in the United States as compared to any other industrialized and wealthy nation. Many commentators have argued forcefully that this structure has been largely responsible for health disparities among minority groups like African Americans who have historically been economically disadvantaged. In the United States, unlike any other industrialized nation, health care is not considered a right for citizens. Thus there has never been a nationalized health care plan, although there has periodically been a good deal of public debate about this.

Few can afford to pay for their own health care out of pocket; thus health insurance is a necessity for almost everyone. While traditionally some form of employer-provided insurance has covered most Americans, in the mid-1960s Medicaid and Medicare were introduced to help cover the unemployed: Medicaid to provide medical coverage for low-income citizens and Medicare to cover senior citizens. These programs were introduced as part of an effort to provide wider health coverage for those who could not afford private insurance to cover their health costs. In theory this has created a two-tiered health care system in which some citizens are covered through private insurance plans and others have some kind of public health care through Medicaid or Medicare plans.

However, to the extent that this coverage ever really worked in reality (which is debatable), it is certainly not working anymore. At the time of this writing, something like a fifth of all Americans lack any health care coverage, while still more are inadequately covered. One problem is that because of the comparatively small amount that Medicaid pays for health services as compared to private health insurance, many private hospitals and physician practices have not accepted Medicaid patients. A second problem that has grown to epidemic proportions concerns the rising numbers of "working poor" or even middle-class people who, though employed, lack any kind of health insurance.

While figures are changing all the time as more and more people lose private health insurance or lose coverage for health benefits they were once entitled to, some relatively recent numbers (from 2000) give a sense of how the economics of health care have played out for African Americans, even during an earlier economic period of relative affluence in the country. At that time, about 56 percent of African Americans had private health insurance while Medicaid covered an additional 22 percent, leaving nearly a quarter uninsured (Kaiser Commission on Medicaid and the Uninsured 2000). The disparity between the number of uninsured whites as compared to African Americans during this period speaks volumes about the way health care is racially distributed.

According to the report put out by the Kaiser Commission: "The uninsured rate for African Americans is more than one and a half times the rate for white Americans, largely because of gaps in employer-based coverage. Although over 8 in 10 African Americans are in working families, employer-sponsored health insurance among African Americans remains substantially lower than that of whites (53% vs. 73%)."

Despite this lack of universal coverage, the United States is also the most expensive health care system among industrialized nations (Mechanic 2008). The costliness of care is primarily due to how it is organized, delivered, and paid for. To follow a very standardized model, health care delivery can be thought of as composed of three sectors: primary (which deals with common sicknesses), secondary (which is hospital based), and tertiary (which handles rare and complex medical conditions requiring the highest levels of technology and the most specialized clinical care). Obviously, each level of care is comparatively more expensive and requires more highly trained and highly paid specialists. Most everyday health problems and preventive care can be addressed by the primary sector in local clinics. In most European countries, the United Kingdom, and Canada (which have nationalized health care), the primary sector is the province of general practitioners and family physicians. It is not hospital based. More than half of the physicians in these countries are trained as general practitioners. Indeed, a few decades ago, most physicians in the United States were also generalists. But things have radically changed in our country, with the vast majority of physicians now specializing. By the beginning of the twenty-first century, the proportion of general physicians had dwindled to about 13 percent, and specialists were treating primary care problems. Not only are specialists more expensive than general or family practitioners, but patients in the United States may have several doctors they see for different health issues, even fairly routine ones like gynecological checkups, that would once have been handled by a single physician.

Access to care in the United States also differs markedly from that in most other countries with nationalized health care plans. In the latter, everyone is assigned a general practitioner as his or her primary doctor. This doctor then makes referrals to specialists if the medical condition of the patient warrants it. In the United States, if a patient can pay (or has insurance to cover costs), that patient can refer him- or herself directly to a specialist and receive high-technology diagnostic tests, thus bypassing the whole first level of primary care. Obviously, this makes health care much more expensive. And indeed costs have skyrocketed over the past several decades. (The cost of health care jumped 70 percent above inflation from the midseventies to the mideighties, just to give an example.)

These burgeoning costs have contributed to the massive increase in the number of Americans who are denied health care because they are not insured. As costs have increased, more and more companies have stopped offering health insurance to their employees. Other economic factors, especially the loss of blue-collar jobs (which tended to be unionized and to include reasonable health care packages) have also contributed to the huge numbers of uninsured. David Mechanic, who has written a great deal about the economics and disparities of health care, offers the following indictment, quoted at length because it so succinctly points out how the structure of care, the costs of care, and the rising numbers of uninsured or underinsured Americans are interconnected:

> Expenditures for services and technologies that many experts believe unnecessary or overused contribute to the high cost of insurance, whether provided through employers, by government, or purchased in the individual market. A significant portion of the population is squeezed out of the market because of these very high costs: about forty-six million people have been uninsured, many more have significant gaps in the continuity of their insurance, and still others have important limitations in their coverage, such as the exclusion of prescription drugs or mental health and substance abuse care. One analysis for the years 2002–2003 estimated that almost one third of those under age sixty-five were uninsured for six months or more. The uninsured are a heterogeneous group by age, employment status, ethnicity, and geography. Yet a majority of those who are uninsured live in a household with an employed member, typically a spouse or parent. Many jobs either do not offer insurance or provide so little financial coverage that what the employee is required to pay to acquire health insurance for the family, or even him- or herself, is not affordable. . . . No other country comes near to spending as much on health care as we do, but all modern nations have developed systems that provide basic coverage for all their citizens. A study of health spending in the United States compared with Organization for Economic Co-Operation and Development (OECD) countries in 2002 found that we spend 53 percent more per capita than Switzerland, the next highest cost country, and 140 percent above median expenditures for all OECD countries. (2008:6)

How do these problems of health coverage affect African Americans more specifically? It is already clear that economics plays an enormous role in quality of care and in health generally. For African Americans, this is a particularly ominous fact because race and class have been so intertwined in this community. African Americans constitute about 13 percent of the U.S. population (American Federation of Labor and Congress of Industrial Organizations [AFL-CIO] 2006). U.S. census data from 2004 to 2006 supply a rough picture of how African Americans are faring as compared to the national average. Most striking, the poverty rate among African Americans is about twice the overall poverty rate (24 percent as compared to 12 percent), and the child poverty rate, though higher in both groups, is also twice that of whites (AFL-CIO 2006). More than a third of African American children live in poverty (34.5 percent) as compared to a national average of about 17 percent (AFL-CIO 2006).

Though Medicaid does cover costs for some of the poorest, it is very incomplete, leaving about 30 percent of those living in poverty without any form of health care (Brodenheimer and Grumbach 2002). This percentage has been increasing over the years as more restrictions have been placed on Medicaid recipients. But extreme poverty is not the only problem for African Americans. Those who are employed (about 60 percent) are also much more likely than whites to be without health insurance (Families USA 2002). (Notably, the Welfare to Work program actually increased this problem, since people were put into low-paying jobs with little or no health care insurance and lost their Medicaid benefits.) Yet another grim statistic is that African Americans working in manufacturing and professional jobs receive about 15 percent less health insurance coverage than whites in the same types of jobs (Families USA 2002). In lower-sector jobs, the difference is even more marked—a 20 percent difference in coverage. African American families with higher incomes remain almost twice as likely as whites to be uninsured (Families USA 2002).

While it is very clear that for the majority of African Americans race and poverty have gone hand in hand, health disparities are not simply an economic or job discrimination issue. Class cannot fully account for poorer health care among blacks. Some research indicates that disparities persist regardless of such markers as social class, education, financial status, or type of health care coverage (M. Good et al. 2002; Dressler 1993). The problem of mistrust persists even among African Americans who are not poor. In our study, even middle-class families have frequently suspected racial profiling in which they were deemed less intelligent or competent because they were black. For example, one parent, herself a nurse, commented,

I think that they're [health professionals] not sure of the intellect they're dealing with . . . even though they all know I'm a nurse. But I think, being the world we do live in, your opinion does not have as much [weight] being black. But that, this is our world.

Medicine and the Construction of Black Identity

Charged moments of suspicion between African American families and clinicians are episodes within a very long history of race and medicine in America. (And if we were to look outside national boundaries, they belong to a global history, a colonization story that spans Europe, Africa, and the Americas.) Perhaps most significant is the rigidly maintained differentiation between blacks and whites that has been central to the formation of America's racial consciousness and its development as a race-based society. The insistence on these dichotomous racial types has meant that being "black" has been defined by any known descent from a black ancestor, creating a particularly inflexible racial category (Smedley 1999). Historically too, "black" has served as an " 'ontological symbol' that is the quintessential signifier of what oppression means in the United States" (Hooks 1992:11). As Goldberg puts it: "Throughout U.S. history, race has always been a central strand of state administration; a silent (and sometimes not so silent) barrier to kinship and adoptability; a condition of advancement and advantage, of power and privilege; and a mark of preference and improvement, of intellectual prowess and jury participation, of law's empire and social injustice, of ethnic excludability and historical denial, of social invisibility and sociospatial segregation. It has been so whether explicitly invoked or silently, invisibly evoked" (1997:10).

Medicine has played a privileged role in the construction of black racial identity (Tapper 1999). Its central place in defining and describing characteristics of black racial identity and bodies belongs to another aspect of American history—the way that "race" itself was marked in the nineteenth century as a specifically scientific term, a term that had legitimacy because it had the weight of scientific knowledge behind it. "Race" was a category within what was then "natural history," what we would now consider biology (Appiah and Gutmann 1996:4).

This is vividly illustrated in records from the post–Civil War period, when physicians "documented" the racial inferiority and anticipated health declines of the newly freed "Negro." "Throughout the nineteenth century the physician remained the chief source of information for comparative race analysis" (Haller 1970:157). Thus, during the country's debates about the legitimacy of slavery, the physical and mental inferiority of blacks (as defended by certain prominent southern physicians) was cited as a cause for the need to keep the institution of slavery alive. Claims were made that freed blacks in the North suffered from idiocy and insanity: "The 1840 U.S. Census 'measured' insanity and idiocy, claiming to show the percentage of blacks suffering both conditions to be greater in the North than in the South. These 'facts' were then used to license the argument that though blacks were at ease with slavery, they were clearly incapable of adjusting to freedom" (Goldberg 1997:38). The role of physicians in the ensuing debate after these statistics were published illustrates how medicine, scientific authenticity, and racial inferiority have influenced America's history. "The argument and the data supposedly supporting it were vigorously challenged by Edward Jarvis, a Massachusetts physician supported by the Massachusetts Medical Society and the American Statistical Association, who demanded that the many miscalculations be formally corrected. Instead, John Calhoun, then Secretary of State and so in charge of the census, censored the critique and persisted in invoking the figures in support of slavery" (Goldberg 1997:38).

Melbourne Tapper uses the example of sickle-cell anemia to explore the intersection of race and medicine in the twentieth century. He argues that "throughout the twentieth century, sickling has emerged and reemerged at the intersection of a variety of medical, genetic, serological, anthropological, personal, and administrative discourses on whiteness, hybridity, tribes and citizenship" (1999:3). He documents how this disease has been deployed to construct black identity through the decades of that century. For example, "During the 1920s, 1930s, and 1940s, medical researchers used sickling to call into question the racial identity of whites afflicted by the phenomenon. From the 1930s through the 1950s, geneticists and anthropologists seized on the disorder to establish the American Negro (as opposed to the black African living in Africa) as a hybrid and therefore inherently diseased individual" (1999:3).

Foucault's discussion of medicine's "pastoral care" (1990) has special salience for those peoples marked as racially inferior, a situation that is, of course, not peculiar to the United States. As Frantz Fanon remarks, while analyzing what he calls "medical supervision" (1963:109), "In the colonial situation, going to see the doctor, the administrator, the constable or the mayor are identical moves" (1963:120). Such visits help administratively to "transform the native into the colonized, self-determining people into colonial or racially marginalized subjects." Medicine thus participates in a "racialized governmentality" (Goldberg 1997:85). One of the most well-known examples of racialized governmentality is the infamous Tuskegee experiment, which was publicly exposed in the early 1970s. This experiment, which involved a forty-year study of untreated syphilis and four hundred black men, is still very much alive in the collective memory of African Americans (Hammonds 1994; Reverby 2000). The response of blacks to its public disclosure is very telling, speaking to the long-standing perception among African Americans that medicine may be used as a racial weapon. "While whites reacted with shock at the exposure of such scientific abuse in their own country . . . , African Americans almost universally saw the study as just one of the more blatant acts of genocide long perpetrated against our communities by whites" (Hammonds 1994:340). The power of this collective memory was evident in our research as well. Families sometimes expressed worry that physicians might be "experimenting on my child." Some refused to take part in our research since it was specifically about African American patients, fearing that it too could be some new version of "Tuskegee."

Families in our study often discussed their fears of racial profiling, but it was rare for clinicians we interviewed to speak in ways that might be considered directly racist or prejudiced. I do not believe this is simply a matter of "covering up" for the researcher. Racism is more insidious than that. Direct racial talk is silenced among clinicians in part because strong moral codes in health care make it difficult for clinicians to consider the possibility that they are drawing upon racial classifications in their dealings with patients. While they may find it perfectly reasonable to recognize differences at an *individual* level, it is highly problematic to speak of difference among *social categories*. As one white doctor put it,

> I don't know that I'm particularly sophisticated about cultural differences. I just try to deal with the families as individuals.

Or as another doctor (also white) said emphatically, "It's the same approach [treatment for everyone]." He explained,

> I'm somewhat lucky in that I grew up in a society that was not . . . uh, so biased, with regards to race . . . I just didn't have preconceived ideas about you know, what black people were like, or what white people were like.

"Othering" tactics practiced by clinicians tend to be subtle and implicit, drawing upon a common taxonomy of terms such as the "noncompliant patient," a language so indirect that its stigmatizing influences go undetected by clinicians themselves (Mattingly and Lawlor n.d.). In our research, negative labels are often affixed to the parents rather than the children themselves. In addition to obvious negative markers—the "abusive, non-compliant or neglectful parent," a language of compassion can serve to create difference: the "overwhelmed parent," the "too many things going on at home parent," the "doesn't really understand the clinical picture" parent, or the "still in denial" parent (Mattingly and Lawlor n.d.).

One of the most insidious features of these categories is that when a person has been placed in one of them, her capabilities and strengths are hidden from view (Lawlor 2004). This problem is exacerbated by the fact that health care encounters are based upon expert models of service delivery—clients have problems, professionals have problem-solving expertise (Lawlor and Mattingly 2009; Mattingly and Lawlor 1998, 2003). This too can make it difficult for professionals to see the need to identify their clients' strong points or to learn from them. In addition to the problematic categories that abound in informal health care discourse, professionals learn narrative strategies that can effectively disguise the abilities of families and children. They work to construct stories that "make sense" of problematic or difficult clients in a way that leaves little room for the patients or families to emerge as agents and to influence the framing of the problem or the path of treatment (Mattingly 1998b).

Issues of trust between clinicians and clients are of particular concern when health conditions are serious and chronic. As I have already suggested, family members are increasingly responsible for providing health care to their children, and the children themselves are asked to carry out "homework" like physical therapy exercises, which requires their cooperation and commitment (Groen, Mattingly, and Meinert 2008). With chronic conditions, there are many chances for things to go wrong. Not only is there no "happy ending" in the form of a cure in sight, but the path of rehabilitation can feel more like one step forward and two steps backward than like any predictable path of progress. This frustrates and frightens patients, families, and clinicians. It also sets up the possibility of blame. If there has not been progress, is someone at fault? Since parents and children are given a great deal of the responsibility for making clinical progress, all parties are potentially culpable. Lack of progress encourages suspicion.

One place this has emerged with startling clarity in our study is with children suffering from sickle-cell disease. The sickle-cell clinic has been the place where race is sometimes openly discussed by clinical staff as well as parents. One mother remarked that children with this disease were "not being treated with dignity and respect" in many hospitals, a lack of respect that included parents as well. Because of some humiliating experiences at the hospital where her child had been a patient for years, she transferred her daughter to another hospital, even though they lacked the same level of expertise in treating sickle-cell disease. She put it this way:

> I'm not a radical. I'm not a feminist . . . I just think you should be treated a certain way, and I should be treated like the person next to me who maybe is a different skin color.

Several clinicians in our study concurred. One physician who had treated sickle-cell patients for twenty-five years and was himself white angrily noted the dismissive way clinical staff tend to view sickle cell, a dismissiveness that also extended to the clinicians who treated children with this "lower-status" disease:

> I'll tell you I don't even listen to them, the attendings. They say, "Ah well, we have a chemotherapy patient coming in so we need to send your sickle patient off the floor because this patient's more important." You know? And I won't tell you what I'd like to say to them . . . There's very much the attitude that, well, this is something that anybody can take care of and it's just like pneumonia. And they don't really believe that there's anything in particular, that special expertise, that's going to help you take care of these kids. And you find out real quick that that's not true.

Problematic, race-based categorizing is revealed in the "med-seeking" label clinicians regularly attach to those with sickle-cell disease who go into a pain crisis. Adolescent African American boys in particular are often refused crucial pain medication or are seen as crazy, violent, or drug seeking when in a pain crisis. The physician quoted above told the following story:

> Try being a seventeen-year-old black male with severe pain going into an emergency room and asking for narcotics and see how far you get . . . Some of the best advice that I ever heard was from an adult with sickle cell, this is from Family Day that we had a few years ago. And this adult said, "What

you need to do is when you're totally fine, you're not in the middle of a crisis, go to the emergency room and ask to meet the head of the emergency room and sit down for five minutes with him and say, 'Hi, my name is blank, remember me? I was an extremist the other night and I'm just on my way to my law firm today, but you know, but on the way to the business I own or the job I have doing X, Y, Z, I wanted to stop in and let you know that I don't always go around in my undershirt and underwear screaming, asking for narcotics.'"

An African American social worker in this same clinic echoed this statement:

As soon as the house staff hears there's a sickle-cell patient, something goes up that says, "I've got a kid here that's drug-seeking, you know, manipulating," without actually doing any assessment of the child.

Learning to "Shuffle and Jive": Acquiring Cultural Competencies to Bridge the Divides

The families in our study sometimes describe their own attempts to get care for their children in strongly marked racial language, implying that they must present themselves as a certain sort of black person in order to get care. It is dangerous to act "loud" or "go ghetto" even when they must protest. If they do find themselves disagreeing with a clinician's opinion, repair work can involve a re-creation of the subservient "Negro," one who knows how to "shuffle and jive." A skill many parents have learned is how to appear less medically competent than they actually are. Parents speak about their need to hide their own expertise when they believe this will threaten clinicians. This is a surprisingly common task, since they are increasingly asked to take on home care that was once the province of clinicians. They need to gain medical competence (such as how to administer a shot) while, at times, taking care to disguise their competencies, which might bring them into conflict with clinicians. On certain occasions, their very expertise may lead them to be categorized as "noncompliant."

One mother describes how she has learned to "shuffle through and play this politicking thing": that is, to *appear* compliant even in situations where she knows more about her child's disease than the professional and may privately disregard what the clinician tells her to do. In situations where she feels she must fight directly, even when she is proved medically correct, she is then faced with yet more "shuffling" and "playing" the "politicking thing" to reestablish good relationships with estranged clinicians. She must, in other words, apologize and act grateful even when she is correct to challenge professionals:

> A lot of times you, as parents you kind of specialize in a disease. You know a lot more than the doctor knows, and it's scary when you have doctors that say, "Oh, I'm Dr. So and So," and . . . then they say something off the wall and you know that they are completely wrong. And how do you deal with a doctor and his ego?

She illustrates this dilemma by telling a story about an escalating confrontation that occurred when she and health professionals disagreed over what was causing her daughter's sudden fever:

> I had a nurse, um, with Betsy. She put in a PICC [peripherally inserted central catheter] line. And in the PICC line, there was a problem with it and my gut told me something was wrong with it. We took her into the ER and they said, "Oh yeah, she has a temperature, there might be something wrong with the PICC. Let's run all these standard tests." And I said, "fine." And then the tests came back that there was no sign of infection in the blood, but she's got this fever. I said, "It's gotta be the PICC line, we just put it in."

The clinicians disagreed, believing her daughter had a viral illness. She replied, "Well, that's fine you think it's a viral illness, you can start her on antibiotics, but don't you think that a doctor should come up and look at the PICC line?" Though the nurses promised that a doctor would come in to check the line, no doctor appeared. The mother watched her daughter's arm swell and became increasingly anxious. With growing intensity, she asked the nurses where the doctor was. They phoned him and he promised to drop by in the morning. At this, the mother snapped:

> Finally, by that time I hadn't had any sleep. I'm anxious, you know. I just look at the nurse and I yell, "Look, I'm not listening to anything you have to say, get out, go get the doctor, and I want him now!" So she runs out of the room. She says, "I'm gonna go get him." She gets the doctor. He comes up twenty minutes later. He looks at it. He says, "Well, we don't want to pull the line." And I said, "I'm not asking you to pull it, I'm asking you to look at it. Run some tests and check it." They check it the next day and, sure enough, it's got a blood clot in it.

She recognized the danger this could have posed to her child and confronted the nurses:

> So I said, "So what would happen if I take my child home and I'm flushing it myself and there's a clot in there and I accidentally push that clot in? What

happens?" "Oh, it could go to her lungs, it could go to her brain, um, you know, the body might absorb it but we don't know. We are going to pull that line."

She might have saved her daughter's life by demanding that the PICC line be checked, but she recognized that she also had set up a situation in which she might appear as a "loud parent" (hence performing a stereotyped "ghetto mom") and thus worried about how to repair her own image and her relationships to the nurses and physicians whose goodwill she desperately needed:

> And by that time, I'm all stressed out, anxious, I feel bad now because I've yelled at the nurse. Now they think, "Oh my God, she's just a really loud parent." And now I go in there, I wonder what these people think of me. I wonder and this is a constant thing . . . it's just this juggling thing of, "Well, you be nice to the nurses so they'll take care of your daughter," but when you assert yourself and say, "Look, I want this and I want this now," what damage have you caused between the relationship that you have with the nurses, the doctors, and everything else? And how are you gonna fix that?

Her solution was to bring in fruit baskets to the hospital staff along with profuse thanks and compliments on their excellent care:

> I take them a big basket and say, you know, "Here you go. You're a great doctor and I love you. You're just great . . . Thank you very much."

If receiving health care involves a kind of game in which one must learn to "shuffle" and play the "politicking thing," there are no guarantees of one's success. Despite this mother's strategic adeptness, over the years a number of the clinical staff grew increasingly hostile to her "interference," and there was even a period where she began taking her daughter to another hospital for treatment because relations with some key staff had become so strained.

THE TALE OF TWO TRAVELERS

In the remainder of this chapter I return to Andrena to portray the ironic aspect of a border travel so riddled with obstacles it often confounds even the most well intentioned and obscures even successful moments of border crossing. I look primarily at two narrative practices, mind reading and storytelling, to consider how border dramas are concretely realized in a clinical setting. I also look at the way race is invoked or implicated in clinical practice even while being hidden by clinicians' invocation of the canonical genres of care.

In this wary space of clinical care such as the one I've been describing, "mind reading" is particularly difficult. Mistakes in narrative mind reading can have disastrous consequences for health outcomes. When clinical interchanges do not go well, it is often because of such misreadings. These charged moments can lead to a spate of aggrieved storytelling by all parties concerned. Even the most minute nuances and gestures of health professionals (especially doctors) can be the subject of much contemplation for families, a subject of storytelling and puzzling. Parents wonder, What are they trying to tell me? What are they hiding? Do they treat me this way because I am black? Because I'm a woman? A man without a job? A single mother? Do they think I'm a "ghetto mom"? Do they think I'm abusing my child? Are they experimenting on my child? Are they refusing care because I'm on public welfare? Do they think I'm not strong enough, bright enough, or educated enough to hear the truth? These are the sorts of questions asked by families in our research, and asked again and again.

No one may want to visit a hospital, especially a big-city hospital, but getting inside is no small feat either. If you are poor, or don't have a doctor who seems very good, your best chance is through the emergency room, where eventually someone has to see you. This was Andrena's usual method in the year before her daughter was finally diagnosed with cancer. When she finally got to the emergency room of this hospital, she was more than determined. She was frantic. The nurse at Belinda's preschool had called three times that week because Belinda was vomiting so violently. "Come and get her," the nurse said. This had been happening for months and months. She'd had to leave work so often to take her daughter to the doctor, or to a hospital emergency room, that finally her boss fired her—regretfully, but she was let go all the same. She had held her job as a receptionist in a car dealership for eleven years and had liked it well enough. More significantly, now that she was unemployed, Andrena lost her health benefits. Now she was on public aid. Meanwhile, her child only got sicker. What could be wrong with her?

I examine some key events in Andrena's encounters with the health care world as these illuminate how narrative (mis)reading and storytelling helped to contribute to "Othering" and to difficulties in getting access to care. I especially look at the role of narrative mind reading and storytelling in constructing difference, and the way that one particular utopian narrative, healing as detective story, is mobilized in these practices. I primarily focus upon two highly charged events centering upon the drama of getting an accurate diagnosis, events that she recounted during that first interview I had with her and returned to over the years in various ways. Hospital staff also discussed these events, though much more obliquely than Andrena's vivid stories did. And they were recorded in a very different language in her daughter's medical chart.

In policy language, these events illustrate dramas of health care access. The first concerns a conflict between Andrena and a doctor in a hospital emergency room. The second concerns a second visit one week later to the same hospital (but a day unit), where Andrena was finally able to get an accurate diagnosis of Belinda. I compare the story that Andrena tells of these two moments with notes from the hospital's medical chart about the same encounters. I explore how actors "read" the minds of their interlocutors, the kind of narrative framings that inform this mind reading and storytelling, and how this serves to produce misunderstandings.

Learning to Fight for Care

In the very first interview with Andrena that I recalled at the start of this book, she launched almost immediately and with very little prompting from me into a harrowing story about her long journey for a diagnosis, an entire year in which she had taken her very sick daughter repeatedly to emergency rooms in hospitals all over the city, only to hear that nothing was seriously wrong with Belinda. A central drama of her story was her mounting fear and frustration as she witnessed her daughter become increasingly ill (with violent vomiting and headaches) while she was sent home again and again after long waits at emergency rooms and other outpatient treatment facilities. Health professionals offered a wide range of advice and possible diagnoses—improper diet or allergies were frequent suspects. Andrena followed these suggestions but nothing helped.

Andrena was at her wits' end. One night there was a particularly violent spate of vomiting. "It was like in *The Exorcist!*" Andrena recalled with a shudder. She rushed Belinda to the emergency room. She recounts the acerbic exchange that followed when the on-call doctor finally saw her daughter. "I had a little confrontation with the lady in

there, okay?" she told me. I asked her to describe what had happened.
Here is the story she told.

> *Andrena:* That evening, when I brought her um—the doctor down there in
> the emergency, she um, came and checked [Belinda], and I was telling
> her, "She's really, she's constantly vomiting and having headaches really
> bad." And she did her little checking, and she said, "Well, I don't see
> anything." And we did her urine and, "I don't see anything." I said, "But
> I'm not leaving here unless you guys tell me to do something because—"
> and then she started, like, getting a little smart on me.
>
> *Cheryl:* Yeah, like what did she say? Just go—just please go through this.
>
> *Andrena:* Okay. She was, like, saying, "Well, if you don't think that I'm
> doing my job, then you could just take her to the, um—I'm gonna make
> you an appointment and you can take her to the day hospital." I said,
> "Oh, it's not that I don't think you're doing your job, I just want my
> daughter to get help." You know, as you understand, I've been taking
> her everywhere and she still be doing the same thing constantly, over and
> over. And so then, she, um—she got a little upset, so she left out—
>
> *Cheryl:* What did she say?
>
> *Andrena:* And she went across the hall and—where her little office was—
> when all that time, the door was open, you know, all the time she was
> seeing patients. But when she left out of there from talking to me, she
> went over there and she closed her door, and I guess she was telling the
> social worker—because the social worker came down and came in there
> and talked to me and was asking me, "What's going on? Is there some-
> thing wrong?" I said, "Yes, there's something wrong." She said, "Well,
> the doctor feels that you don't think she's doing her job." I said, "So,
> but why does she have to call the social worker on me?" You know?
> And then I started feeling like they was, um—I felt like she thought that
> I was, like, kind of crazy or did something to my daughter myself. That's
> the kind of feeling I had got. I felt kinda—very uncomfortable. I said,
> "Do you guys call the social worker on *all* people?" You know? And
> she—and I was letting the social worker explain. "No, it's not on all
> people. It's just when the parents feel that you're not happy with your
> doctor, and the doctor will call." You know, but then, she kinda calmed
> me down. You know, I wasn't arguing or I wasn't saying any, you know,
> bad—anything—I just wanted my baby to get help, you know? I didn't
> want to take her home again and be like she was. You know, she'd done
> been through it too much.

In Andrena's story, the doctor's fear of Andrena played a part in
preventing her from listening in detail to Andrena's description of Belinda's worsening symptoms. Andrena got the "uncomfortable feeling"
that the doctor saw her as "kind of crazy" and was even suspicious
that Andrena had hurt her own daughter. Andrena herself said that by

the time she got to the emergency room on this visit, she "was going crazy" with worry. It is not difficult to imagine that an emergency room doctor could attribute Andrena's panic and refusal to accept her diagnosis (nothing is medically wrong) to a mother's precarious mental state, or worse, to her being an abusive parent. City emergency rooms in the middle of the night get their quota of the mentally unstable. Furthermore, health professionals, like everyone else in contemporary America, are on the alert for parent-child abuse.

From Andrena's standpoint, the exchange with the emergency room doctor was a turning point. In her tale, it figures as a key episode in a plot that underscores the moral necessity of noncompliance. Access sometimes even requires trespassing, as can be heard in the next episode of her story. A week later, as she recounted, she returned to the hospital with an even sicker child. The hospital receptionist told her to come back a month later at her appointed date. This time Andrena resisted in a more active way. She looked past the reception desk to a door that, Andrena said, had a sign "The Administrator." (In fact, there is no such ominous sign.) Behind this door was a suite of offices of doctors and secretarial staff, whom she had often seen coming and going. This space was off limits to patients and families. Andrena picked Belinda up in her arms, marched past the protesting receptionist and through the suite of rooms, declaring to the startled secretaries, "My baby is sick. She needs help and I'm not leaving until somebody sees my baby!" A doctor was summoned. He asked Belinda to tell him where it hurt. Belinda pointed to the back of her head. He asked her to walk. She did, wobbling to one side. He ran for another doctor and they asked her to walk again. Again she wove, listing to her right. Two days later, Belinda had a CAT (computerized axial topography) scan and a subsequent diagnosis of a malignant brain tumor that had grown, Andrena remembers, to "the size of an egg." Andrena was told the tumor had been growing unchecked for at least a year. Prognosis was poor.

Diagnostic Puzzles: The View from the Medical Record

I now turn to Belinda's medical record to glean something of the health professionals' perspectives on these events. Though sketchy, the chart notes are remarkably telling. They corroborate Andrena's version of events and yet suppress the moral connections made in Andrena's account. Here is an excerpt from the emergency room doctor's notes about their charged interaction. "Vague history of complaint . . . normal gait . . . social problems . . . ref to social work . . . Diagnosis: vomiting, psychosocial concerns, parent-child conflict." We hear nothing of a confrontation, but there is an ominous suggestion about Andrena's emotional state and her possible fitness as a mother. Intriguingly, a conflict is reported, but it is portrayed as occurring between parent and child rather than between parent and doctor. There is also a note by the social worker, the one "called on," who mentions in more sympathetic tones the mother's "frustration and fear."

Andrena's story of her confrontation with the emergency room doctor, coupled with the doctor's notes in the medical chart, offers an eloquent instance of Andrena's "narrative mind reading." Just as Andrena feared, the doctor saw her as a possibly abusive mother. Andrena "read" the doctor's mind with acuteness. She told me, "And then I started feeling like they was, I felt like she thought that I was, like, kind of crazy or did something to my daughter myself." Her capacity to do such mind reading is a matter of reading public symbols. The arrival of the social worker, the doctor's closing her office door that had been open earlier, these overt behaviors were accurately read by Andrena as signs that her protests had placed her in the dangerous category of "problem parent," perhaps even "abusive parent." Or, as the emergency doctor wrote in the medical chart, Andrena's behavior indicated the presence of "psychosocial concerns" and "parent-child conflict."

This ability to read the doctor's mind depends upon a domain of culturally shared understandings about what should happen in an emergency room encounter. Most obviously, emergency rooms are supposed to be for *emergencies,* not routine medical care. Andrena did not seem to have an emergency, as far as the doctor could ascertain, and therefore had no proper place in this setting, no right to take up any more of the doctor's time. Through her frantic insistence, Andrena violated the code of proper parent behavior. This charged encounter also reveals what happens in border zones when meanings are only partly shared and where interlocutors perceive one another as Other. Andrena could not find a way to convey that she was a very concerned parent with a truly ill child. She was African American and was in the emergency room, a place in which a major role of the doctor is to "get rid" of all those parents who bring their children in for routine problems, thus glutting the system with nonemergencies.[7]

The very next entry in the medical chart comes six days later, written by the doctor Belinda saw after Andrena had carried her into the administrative offices. This was the doctor who recognized that Belinda was probably seriously ill. His report does not mention Andrena's unorthodox trespass into the doctors' quarters. Instead, his entry indicates, along with some general description of the symptoms described by Andrena, the possibility of a brain tumor. He notes that a CAT scan has been ordered: "Phys Exam: looks well but wobbly . . . has me concerned about mass in head, will schedule CT." A further entry, three days later, reports that Belinda has had surgery. The neurosurgeon states in the record that they did a "partial resection with VP shunt placement." There is also a note by the hospital chaplain from that same day stating he has met with the family to offer "spiritual support."

The most important feature of these terse notes is what is missing. This is a genre of narrative (if one wishes to call it that) notable for its significant absences. To follow Aristotle's (1967) idea that stories offer moral arguments through the organizing function of the plot, the medical chart "narrative" denies the moral that Andrena's story makes. It does so not by offering a counterargument, a counterplot, but by producing a kind of flattening of narrative. It appears to organize events as a series, a "chronicle," in Hayden White's terms (1980, 1987). A chronicle places events in a chronology; it is structured as a series. It recounts events in such a truncated way that it obscures rather than illuminates what is central to the way actions are linked to motives as well as to consequences. Ochs and Capps, following Heath, also distinguish chronological accounts of actions (Heath calls them recasts) from emplotted narratives. "Recasts are logically simple in that they do not center around a breach of expectations nor do they link events into a plot structure" (2001:85). Referring to oral discourse, they note that recasts "tend to be grammatically, lexically, and phonologically relatively flat" (2001:85). This is also an apt description of written medical records.

Narratively speaking, Andrena's story is much richer than the chart notes. Notably, it contains the kind of well-developed causal argument that comes with a narrative plot, one where actions suggest motives and intentions and lead compellingly to consequences. In her tale, doctors' refusals to take her seriously result in repeated misdiagnoses of her daughter's condition, and when a diagnosis is finally made—significantly only after she has caused what Kenneth Burke would call Trouble—her daughter is very ill with advanced cancer. For a long time Andrena wondered whether her daughter would still be alive if she had been able to get the attention of the doctors sooner. By contrast, the clinic gaze, as instantiated through the medical charts, reveals another kind of narrative strategy, an institutionalized insistence on chronicle rather than narrative proper. In the records, Andrena's charged encounter with the emergency room doctor is reduced to an isolated instance that (evidently) has no bearing on, and does not bear upon, the events that are later recorded. No clinician narrator returns to the medical record to emplot the earlier episodes in an unfolding history, to reread the past in light of what later unfolds.

The Narrative Production of Border Conflict: Violations of a Healing Genre

Narrative mind reading and storytelling play a critical part in the rocky relationship between this mother and the health professionals. In the emergency room conflict, the doctor, as portrayed through both Andrena's story and her own chart notes, defines Andrena in a particular way because Andrena does not play her part properly. The doctor quickly (if erroneously) interprets Andrena's intentions because she relies upon a canonical genre, in this case the detective story, to understand how "emergency room" encounters ought to unfold, what the roles of the various characters (like patients and families) are, and what kinds of actions characters ought to take in order to further this dramatic plot in a proper and efficacious manner. While sometimes border conflicts arise because families and clinicians do *not* share the same dramatic healing genre, this is not true here. The doctor and Andrena are not in conflict over *which* dramatic genre is correct; this physician acts in a way that implicitly presumes she is in charge of identifying when a serious medical mystery presents itself. This is exactly what Andrena hopes she will do. The implicit and utopian character of this dramatic genre is obvious if you consider what the doctor *cannot* say (probably even to herself). She cannot say, "I believe your daughter may be very ill, but we are not going to explore this further because tests are expensive and you are on public aid." Instead, as her chart notes indicate, the doctor tacitly reaffirms that she *would* do better detective work if the situation warranted it, but since it does not, any fault must lie with the parent.

The wariness of actors within this border space encourages the construction of well-known plots that concern typical violations. The power of these plots makes it difficult for actors to transcend their assigned roles. Even breaches become conventionalized. Despite this conventionality, it is too simple to see this cultural Othering as the result of automatic and nondeliberative prejudgments. The conflict precipitated by the emergency room doctor's behavior is not because the doctor dismisses Andrena out of hand from the start. Though she sees no obvious observable signs of a serious medical problem, she does run some lab tests. It is when these too come back negative that Andrena acts upon a significantly different narrative—what might be called a "breach story" (Amsterdam and Bruner 2000).

What is being "breached" here? One of the most canonical dramatic genres—the detective story. Andrena is not able to present a significant "medical mystery" to the doctor. Obviously, this is not Andrena's fault. In an emergency room it is particularly necessary to be able to present oneself either with a definite, even life-threatening medical condition or, at the least, with an extremely serious and mysterious set of symptoms that demand further investigation. Vague, chronic symptoms are unlikely candidates, especially in an emergency room, to signal a medical mystery that requires detective work on the part of clinicians. But this, in itself, does not constitute a breach. Rather, it is Andrena's *insistence* that violates one of the key assumptions of this canonical genre, namely, that it is the patient who comes with the mystery and the doctor who is the detective.

This assumption is, of course, an especially idealized one. Commonly, it is the patients or family members who function as the initial detectives. When symptoms are recurrent and intransigent in the face of a variety of treatments, as in Belinda's situation, what initially seems like a minor problem turns into a full-blown mystery. For Andrena, Belinda's illness has been transformed from something worrisome into a true horror story of *Exorcist* proportions; her child is under attack by a dangerous but unknown criminal. But Andrena cannot convey this to a physician, who has not lived through her experience and who is disinclined to believe her without any corroboration from her own examination. It is not part of the canonical tale that the patient (or the patient's family) serves as co-detective. And in this dramatic genre it is the body's symptoms and signs, not patient reports, that are supposed to lead clinicians to suspect not only a crime but the probable identity of the criminal. From the doctor's perspective, if any crime is being committed, it is this difficult parent who is the culprit.

"Familiar Stranger" Stories

Breach stories help to further the construction of the cultural Other in an especially powerful way. In stories, characters are created. Or, as Aristotle (1967) put it, narratives concern "men in action." They are as much about the "men" as about the action. Aristotle argued that stories reveal characters through the actions they take. What kind of character is created in stories like Andrena's? In narratives like hers that recount dramatic clinical encounters across racial, class, and professional divides, narrative trouble is not precipitated by the *mysteriousness* of the foreigner. Rather, the trouble upon which the plot turns comes from the problematic actions of a "familiar stranger." A troublesome familiar stranger is the sort of character whose actions are predictable but unreasonable, unaccountable, deeply flawed, possibly immoral. Narrative mind reading is possible because actors draw upon a familiar stock of stories across a vast range of situations. In familiar stranger encounters, actors depend upon well-developed culturally based notions of what various kinds of Others are likely to be up to and what their motivations (however, unreasonable, flawed, etc.) probably are. One mark of familiar stranger stories is the anonymity assigned to the Other. In Andrena's story, for instance, we have "the doctor" rather than a doctor with a particular name. Characters in the story (social workers, receptionists, nurses and doctors) are depicted in stereotypical terms.

Most compelling, however, is the way Andrena's story reveals how she sees herself as designated by the doctor. When Andrena realizes that the doctor has not only left but also *closed her door,* a door that "all that time . . . was open," the doctor is represented as not only hostile but fearful of Andrena. When she does not return but sends out a social worker instead, this only confirms to Andrena that she has come to be seen as possibly dangerous. Calling upon a social worker has a very special meaning in such a context. For many underclass African American families, social workers connote trouble. Operating as a kind of hospital police force, they signal a particular reading of the client's character. Andrena's account communicates her own double bind. If she is to try to get care for her daughter, she is forced to act in such a way that she appears to the (mostly white, overwhelmingly middle-class) doctors as a menacing person. In a different context, the psychiatrist Frantz Fanon offers a powerful allegory of such an experience, remembering his first terrifying trip to France from his homeland of

Martinique in the 1950s. "'Mama, see the Negro! I'm frightened!'" a little white girl cries to her mother. "Frightened," he continues, amazed. "Now they were beginning to be afraid of me. I made up my mind to laugh myself to tears, but laughter had become impossible" (1963:112). Andrena's story, though lacking Fanon's dark irony, echoes his anguish, portraying what it is like to be designated as an Other, a person who, needing help that is repeatedly denied, comes to be fixed as a person who menaces.

Despite the marked difference in narrative style and genre between Andrena's rich narrative and the chart notes, there is an important similarity between the two accounts. Both offer familiar stranger stories. What Andrena's account shares with the medical record is a flat rendering of the Other. The distinction in literary theory between "flat" characters and round ones is helpful here. E.M. Forster tells us that flat characters, in their purest form, are "constructed round a single idea or quality" (1927:67). Once they are identified, flat characters never surprise us, never waver. They do exactly what they are supposed to do, no more and no less. A flat character, Forster notes, can be described in a single sentence. " 'I will never desert Mr. Micawber.' There is Mrs. Micawber—she says she won't desert Mr. Micawber, she doesn't, and there she is" (1927:68). Round characters, by contrast, possess multiple qualities, shadowy ambiguities, and outright contradictions. Most important, they are capable of change.

The type of "stories" told in clinical charts supports a flat rendering of characters through its selectivity as well as the comparative absence of plot. As clinicians say, to decipher stories in a medical chart you must learn to "read between the lines." Medical charts recount small moments here and there. These highly abbreviated short stories, multiply authored, are strung along, one after the other, as separate entries in the record without being woven into a coherent plot. Chart reporting supports an episodic structure in which events take their place and have their meaning as a succession of "nows" rather than the complex temporality that characterizes fuller narratives. This manner of speaking fits a "manner of operating," as de Certeau (1984) puts it. It assists in keeping the professional clinical gaze in place. It does not challenge the canonical narratives or their claims to an objective view, for it leaves no official room for guilt. This guiltlessness is facilitated because in a simplified chronicle connections between earlier actions and subsequent consequences are not compellingly drawn. In Andrena's case, this means that the chart record does not support any recognition of the unending misdiagnoses she and her daughter have endured. And because of this, it does not provide a "reading" of Andrena's mind that facilitates accurate interpretations of Andrena's subsequent behavior with health professionals, including her wariness of what health professionals tell her and her minor acts of resistance.

Cultural borderlands as zones of friction are narratively furthered by storytelling strategies that paint characters in this flat way. Stories peopled with flat characters help to make predictable certain kinds of relationships, even those stabilized around conflict. Such characters can be just as useful to the everyday storyteller (a clinician, a patient, a family caregiver) as they are to the novelist, for they do not confuse the "point" of the story by introducing moral complexities and unexpected turns of the plot. "It is a convenience for an author when he can strike with his full force at once, and flat characters are very useful to him, since they never need reintroducing, never run away, have not to be watched for development, and provide their own atmosphere— little luminous disks of a pre-arranged size, pushed hither and thither like counters across the void or between the stars; most satisfactory" (Forster 1927:69). When health professionals and their clients portray one another as flat characters, they have much more control over the plot and the moral of the story; characters need not be "watched for development." Once narratively fixed, their actions and motives gain transparency, and they can be quickly reckoned with as predictable causes for outcomes. Since actual humans are not flat, narratives that portray them in this way can be told only if there are discursive strategies that allow "real-life" storytellers to ignore a great deal of what is actually done and said.

Reinforcing Border Conflict: The Social Life of Stories

Stories are more than texts and do more than reconstruct past events; they shape the meaning of the present and anticipate the future. Andrena has retold her story a half-dozen times during subsequent interviews. It has plainly haunted her. It has played a pivotal role in her ongoing construction of the clinical world as a treacherous place, necessary for survival but filled with danger. Andrena's story, or part of it, traveled to other parents in the clinic. In past years, I have heard Andrena tell versions of it not only to me but also to other parents and family caregivers who have ill children. After Belinda had surgery, Andrena stayed with her in the hospital, usually on the east wing. There she got to know other parents whose children also had cancer. They shared stories of their struggle to get a diagnosis and their repeated trips to emergency rooms. Some told stories like Andrena's. Swapping "horror stories" takes on a political dimension, binding together families whose troubled experiences with health care emerge as a shared problem rather than an idiosyncratic experience. It has also brought some relief to Andrena, for if she is not alone, then the delayed diagnosis was not so clearly her fault. She need not shoulder so much blame for her compliance—that is, for allowing herself to obey the "doctor's orders" for an entire year while her daughter's tumor grew unchecked. This storytelling, coupled with her own experience, reinforced Andrena's conviction that it was important to learn how to be noncompliant, a "just-right noncompliance" that was a difficult skill to learn. It required the cultivation of numerous deceptions and devious maneuvers, what Scott (1985) and de Certeau (1984) have famously labeled "weapons of the weak."

A different version of her story circulated among some of the clinical staff that treated Belinda. As I came to interview Belinda's rehabilitation therapists, I discovered that Andrena had also told truncated versions of this story to some of them, for when I asked them how Belinda had entered treatment, a few noted that Andrena had told them it had taken many months to get a proper diagnosis. None ever mentioned the defiant act that had finally produced a new "clinical gaze" and from there a new diagnosis. Perhaps Andrena never told them. The clinicians I interviewed consistently narrated a history of Andrena's repeated and frustrated visits to doctors and emergency rooms without obtaining a diagnosis. They mentioned that this had been a long process. But they never recounted the two key events in the story Andrena told me—the confrontation with their hospital's emergency room doctor, and the drama of her trespass through the doors of "The Administrator" that finally led to a diagnosis. Their stories, like Andrena's, portrayed Andrena as a victim of a long process of delayed diagnosis but *lacked* an account of the events that had led to treatment. That is, their versions never connected Andrena's difficulties accessing health care to her subsequent noncompliance, precisely the moral that Andrena's story highlights.

There were other differences in the stories the clinicians told. While Andrena recounted her story with fervor, the therapists repeated it furtively, lowering their voices uneasily as they told me what they had heard. The agonizing year of waiting with a sicker and sicker child while being given repeated misdiagnoses was inevitably foreshortened in their versions to "several months." This was not a story they were fond of telling; narrations were cursory and vague. "I think she said maybe four or five months before she got a diagnosis," they would say. "It must have been pretty hard for her."

Andrena's story offers a hard lesson about what it means to be the parent of a seriously ill child, namely that compliance can be a terrible thing. Clinicians did not participate in this story line. For them, her subsequent minor acts of insurrection were not episodes within a "horror story" in which noncompliance was necessary to get health care. Instead, their version supported a view that Andrena was not a very compliant parent. They turned to another familiar story to explain this—the "home problems" narrative, in which they attributed her behavior not to hard-won wisdom but to being "overwhelmed." This, in turn, they ascribed to problems "at home," especially the breakup of her marriage. They "read" Andrena's mind in ways that emplotted her actions as episodes in an often-told tale concerning poor, African American women. Andrena became a protagonist in a story of family struggles, missing husbands, poverty, and other social ills that confronted her with immense challenges and made it difficult for her to collaborate properly with health professionals.

This prototypical tale is, in some respects, perfectly accurate. It is indeed true that women like Andrena routinely face enormous economic and social problems while trying to care for their ill children. Husbands often are not there for them. But this story misses the most important events that have shaped Andrena's response to the health professionals who treat Belinda. This narrative of a difficult home life is disconnected in the professionals' stories from the role of health care practice in compounding her troubles. The "home problems" narrative provides a script for the emergency room doctor who is unable to find something medically wrong with Belinda in her cursory examination. The nurses Andrena argues with rely upon it, especially when they find Andrena has too many visitors in Belinda's hospital room or does not sufficiently discipline her daughter. And it is employed by the occupational and physical therapists who are continually dismayed to find that Andrena does not sit in the waiting room during outpatient physical and occupational therapy appointments but instead "disappears" until the sessions are over.

As we can see, such storytelling can also play a powerful role in creating new communities, ones that help to reinforce border conflicts of an "us-them" mentality. This has been especially true for families in the study who say again and again that caring for a child with a serious illness has forced them to create relationships with other families who are facing the same troubles. This besieged community building among patients (or families) is a powerfully recurring theme.

The Circulation of Dystopic Stories

Andrena's story of her emergency room conflict is nested within a larger narrative about contemporary health practices that violate ethical medical behavior. This is a violation of the canonical dramatic genres that are *supposed* to govern everyday practice. These clinical genres share the (utopian) assumption that hospitals exist for clinicians to diagnose and treat sick people rather than to turn them away or compel parents to break the rules in order to get care for their children. Families, too, share these cultural narratives in their belief that they *ought* to be entitled to care when their children are very sick and must be taken to the emergency room. When, in actuality, this dramatic expectation fails so utterly, such failure serves as fertile ground for stories that document the inhumanity of care. Andrena's account suggests her own impossible position as a person who must choose between not being a good mother by obeying the doctor (and therefore taking a sick child home again) or not being a good mother in the eyes of the hospital staff and thus possibly jeopardizing future health care for her child at one of the best hospitals in the city. Thus her story points toward a breach at a societal level.

Dystopic pictures of clinical practice and clinical hope are very compelling in capturing what goes so terribly wrong here. Health emerges as a kind of Hobbesian war of each against each, or a Bourdieu-like competitive game in which "prizes" like basic health care are withheld from those who lack the symbolic capital to win them. Clinicians routinely invoke this imagery when they wonder whether a patient is "worthy" of care. Should they allocate the resources of their own time or of expensive medical procedures to a particular patient? In this competition, health is a scarce resource that is available only to those who "win" it versus those who must inevitably lose. This kind of cost-benefit decision making is a routine part of care, one that American clinicians, at any rate, cannot avoid. It is so routine, in fact, that it hardly seems to have any dramatic structure to it at all, except as we see it played out "on the ground" by someone like Andrena.

Foucault's dystopia of healing as incarceration, a drama of discipline and punishment, is also present as Andrena is pulled aside by the social worker who functions as a kind of prison guard. While in a general sense these dystopic portraits describe the everyday business of clinical care, they emerge as *central* dramas of care for the actors themselves— especially for the families—when the utopian genres fail. Clinicians, too, sometimes complain that they have become gatekeepers for scarce resources or jailors of "noncompliant" patients, roles they never intended to play when they entered medicine and ones that make it very difficult for them to sustain and nurture their vision of themselves as healers.

Andrena's story hints at the way dystopic dramas are reinvented and reproduced in everyday practice. Her experience of the emergency room, coupled with other experiences she has had in trying to seek care for her daughter—especially the full year of fruitless trips to hospital emergency rooms throughout the city—is narrated and renarrated to other parents, who have similar stories of their own. For Andrena and many other parents, such powerful experiences, meriting powerful stories, are pivotal to the production of an inhumane drama peopled by uncaring, inattentive, or incompetent health professionals. In response, such stories suggest that families devise their own strategic maneuvers to counter professional dismissiveness, trying to learn how to act out a "just-right" noncompliance to get care for their children. As we can already see, practices of surveillance and punishment not only accompany health care but may be intensified if clinicians perceive that the "scarce resource" of health is not being well used, owing to "noncompliant" patients and parental caregivers.

But these dystopic lessons are not the only ones to be drawn from Andrena's narration. She also recounts a story of successful resistance. She "trespasses," and through this transgression into forbidden hospital territory she does finally get attention for her daughter. On the one hand, this is the good news—there is some possibility for action, some chance to get an institution as monolithic as a large urban hospital to pay attention. And this is a possibility even if one not only is poor and black but also has already been "written up" in the charts as a problem parent. But this possibility for action, for transforming a situation and engendering the canonical drama she has been pleading for (the detective story in which a doctor finally takes charge and promises to do a thorough investigation until the criminal has been found), also introduces vulnerability, including ethical vulnerability. Andrena must ask herself, Was she truly a good parent if she was unwilling to take the risk of defying the health care system before her daughter got so sick? Did she truly leave every stone unturned? Why was she so compliant for so long?

The chance to act in a transformative way also opens up a space of hope. Even upon hearing the horrifying news of just how sick her daughter is, she sees the beginnings of other possible actions that have transformation potential. This includes learning new skills of being defiant enough to try to get care without getting rejected altogether. It also includes reaching out and teaching and learning from other parents who have faced similar difficulties and are also forced to learn new skills of border crossing and border transgressing.

Andrena's acts of defiance and the terrible diagnosis that follows stand as an episode in a new kind of acted story, one that I will trace throughout this book and especially return to in my final chapters. This is a moral journey she embarks upon where she must struggle with how to hope in new ways, undergoing the dramatic task of changing herself so that she can travel down a road as desperate as the one she now faces.

CHAPTER 4

Widening the Gap

The Creation of a Conflict Drama

When a contentious relationship has emerged and embattled interlocutors have been designated by one another as troublesome familiar strangers, it is extremely difficult to circumvent conflicts or challenge these powerful designations. The case that follows reveals the struggles between a father (Ron) and a physical therapy aide (Marcia) in which the father has already been prefigured by much of the clinical staff as a "noncompliant dad" who "does not step up to the plate" in caring for his very ill daughter suffering from sickle-cell disease.

What is especially interesting in this case is not the struggle itself, which is common enough, but how this father's familiar stranger designation is produced so inexorably despite several factors that might have challenged it, including a deeply felt shared concern by both aide and father that his very sick daughter be able to walk again and leave the confines of her wheelchair. Their manner of relating to one another easily disguises this mutual desire. In fact, both at times can appear indifferent or even outright callous toward the child. In the interaction, the aide emerges as another kind of familiar stranger dreaded by parents, the "uncaring clinician" who is "just there to do her job." How is it that their heartfelt concerns for the child are so invisible to one another? How do they fail to see their shared commitments? What I try to show is that they came to the session with such profound mutual misunderstanding of one another partly because the healing genres that shape their narrative expectations of what *should* unfold in a session are very different.

Ron reflects a widespread family perspective. Families caring for chronically ill or disabled children generally participate with clinicians in the same aspirations that the biomedical genres embody: the hope of detecting causes, of making repairs, of beating the disease, of finding a cure. However, families are often, and of necessity, more compelled than clinicians by the problems of how to manage everyday life when none of these canonical hopes are fulfilled. It is not surprising that, again and again, families express their strongest allegiance to the genre of healing as transformative journey, recognizing that they and their children must change in profound ways simply to manage the illness or disability. More significantly, they must change in order to avoid despair, a threat parents frequently worry about. Thus parents embark on a *quest* for hope and undertake the difficult moral work of sustaining and cultivating this quest.

Clinicians, by contrast, generally foreground the biomedical genres; these are governed by ideals of measurable efficacy, competence, and scientific knowledge. Clinicians often recognize that patients and families must undertake a transformative journey of some kind, but they tend to believe that compliance with the duties and obligations imposed by the canonical genres (and the experts) provides the key to this transformative task. Patients and patients' caregivers must change, in other words, in order to comply. But parents tend to develop a long-term and broad sweeping picture of the metamorphosis that is required, one that sometimes takes them far from the demands of clinical compliance. It is this difference in perspective that helps to produce the conflictual drama between aide and father that I recount below.

The clinical session I will describe is preceded by a family fight that erupts unexpectedly in the hospital room where Ron's daughter, Ronetta, is staying. This skirmish between Ron and his ex-wife plays a crucial role in shaping the difficulties of the subsequent clinical session, so I begin there.

THE FAMILY FIGHT

When Ron walks into his daughter's hospital room, he sees that she is nauseous again. She begins to vomit. He quickly grabs a small bedpan to put under her mouth, trying to comfort her. "Cough it up," he says gently as he strokes her forehead. She sobs: "This is too much work. I just want someone to put me out of my misery." He quietly hushes her, sighing. Ronetta has sickle-cell anemia, and it is so severe she has already had a stroke. Now she is in a wheelchair, having to learn how to walk all over again. She is only twelve years old.

As Ron stands in the room, stroking his daughter's head and struggling with how to comfort her, Ronetta's mother, Rena, suddenly enters, accompanied by a church lady friend. Hasn't the hospital staff forbidden Rena to come? Ron turns away when Rena challenges him, asking him where he has been. Without replying, he walks out of the room and goes downstairs for a cigarette to "cool off." When he returns a few minutes later, Rena and her friend are still there. Rena again confronts him.

> *Rena:* Ronetta feels like we don't love her. You are never here, and I can't stay overnight. She sees all these other kids with parents here all the time. I should be able to stay overnight with her.

(The hospital staff shares Ron's view that Rena is an "unfit mother" and has placed a visitation restriction on her. She is not allowed any overnight visits.)

> *Ron:* She's not a five- or six-year-old. You don't *need* to be here overnight.
>
> *Rena:* I know I don't *need* to. I want to.
>
> *Rena's friend:* Put yourself in the other person's shoes. Wouldn't you want to come visit her?
>
> *Ron: (muttering to himself)* Put myself in the other shoes: you can *have* her, but you have to get your act together first.
>
> *Rena: (voice rising)* All this is happening because of *you*. God has told me that we need to be here with her.
>
> *Ron: (retorting angrily)* I come here, but I can't be here for her 100 percent of the time.
>
> *Rena:* They do horrible things to her when you're not around. A nurse told me that they stuck a tube up her nose, and she was just sitting in her chair, leaning forward, just crying. They don't treat her as good as they would if we were here.
>
> *Ron: (shouting)* I don't have to listen to this.
>
> *Rena's friend: (speaking up, admonishing both of them)* Listen, just calm down and think about this. Maybe you should just talk about it another time. Just pray about it and talk later.

Ron angrily stalks out of the room. A few minutes later Rena leaves. Ron returns again, sitting quietly with Ronetta while waiting for the physical therapist. His expression is grim.

Ron has come to the hospital that day primarily because the reha-bilitation team has asked him to attend some "family training sessions" so that he can learn therapy programs they expect him to carry out at home with his daughter once she is discharged. He is having trouble with many of the staff. "These folks have been ripping and running," he complains, barraging him with more and more forms so that he is constantly "signing this and signing that." They are always taking him by surprise. "And they come at me when I'm least expecting it. And it's like everything they suggest, or have an idea about, they want me to agree with it." Many things they suggest make "a lot of sense," and he goes ahead and "signs" or "agrees with" them to some degree. But in his view, the staff does not extend him the same courtesy that he gives them. They do not seem to try to understand the situation from his point of view. As he puts it: "Sometimes it's just, it's where they want *me* to see what *they* see, but *they* don't want to see what *I* see."

Ron has a new wife and a baby boy, and his new wife is not enthu-siastic about stepping in to care for Ronetta. It is really up to him. And all this has happened so quickly. A few months earlier he was given custody of his terribly ill daughter because his ex-wife, suffering from schizophrenia, was no longer deemed a fit parent. This unfitness was not simply due to her mental instability, but also due to her religious beliefs that meant she was unwilling to follow prescribed medical treat-ments for her child. Rather than see her enter foster care, her father took custody of Ronetta. His life changed overnight. Not only did he have a new wife and child, but he was trying to look after his ailing mother. He was only sporadically involved in Ronetta's life before this change of custody. He hates having Ronetta spend months at a time in the hospital, but he also does not see how he can manage all this care at home. As he puts it while thinking over the staff's attitude toward him:

> When the time comes for Ronetta to go home, they [the staff] gonna tell me that she can't come home unless I complete these here therapy sessions. Which is okay. I don't mind doing what I can. But, you know, I'm no thera-pist. I don't really know what to do, or how to do certain things with her . . . And then they try to put that weight on me and make, like, well, if I don't do this, then I'm abandoning her. That's not true. That's not so. God knows I've been, I've stood by Ronetta through thick and thin, from the time they took her from her mom. And it's been only me.

The hardest thing for Ron, though, is his daughter's depression and despair. Ronetta has asked to be put out of her misery more than once.

"I can't believe Ronetta is talking about dying," Ron remarks shaking his head in near-defeat. And her mother—his ex-wife—isn't helping any, in his view. She is a deeply religious Jehovah's Witness, and he fears her influence over Ronetta.

> You know, her mom always talks about "The Rapture." That's what Ronetta is doing. She's waiting for "The Rapture" to take her away from this pain.

How can he persuade her to continue to live with her pain and disability? "She needs to learn that it's not going to be easy, but she can't just give up! You know," he adds, "when you are depressed, your body deteriorates too. That's what is happening to Ronetta."

Marcia is the physical therapy aide assigned to do the training with Ron. She has treated Ronetta often and she knows Ron a little. She tried to do this training with him once before and it did not go well. Some of the staff, like Dr. Morten, Ronetta's hematologist and head of the sickle-cell team, defend Ron. But Marcia shares the view, along with most of the nurses and therapists in the unit, that Ron is not "stepping up to the plate." He isn't there for his daughter "through thick and thin," she says, eerily echoing Ron's own phrasing as he defended his behavior. "I think he means well," she concedes reluctantly, "but his mind is somewhere else. I think he cares about her [Ronetta], but he doesn't care about all those dirty little steps of fatherhood where you have to be there through thick and thin. You always have to be there. You can't go out and feel like you have to do your own thing because your kids need you right now."

Marcia finds it difficult to work with him because he never seems to listen. "I try to tell him how to do things and he just says the opposite when I'm training him," she complains. When she has told him that his daughter was capable of doing many things herself, he has disagreed. " 'I'm just gonna lift her anyways.' " She has tried to explain to him that he does not need to help Ronetta in that way. "Ronetta does as much as she can, because she's capable of this, this, and this. 'You don't have to lift her. She can do this.' But it's like, he can't hear it," she concludes in frustration.

We can hear her irritation from the moment Marcia walks into Ronetta's room to begin the training session that I will describe below. She has already heard from one of the nurses that Ron and Rena have had a big fight. There has been a "big blowout," people have told her, and Ronetta is in her room crying. This does not bode well. But from Marcia's perspective these home exercises have to be done.

Otherwise, Ronetta may have to be put into foster care for her own good. This is an option the staff have been discussing in team meetings for some time.

NARRATIVE PREFIGURING: THE MISUNDERSTANDING OF UNDERSTANDING

With remarkable synchrony, both Ron and Marcia enter the family training session filled with dread that they are heading into battle, their good intentions and concerns invisible to the other. Their dread goes far beyond any personal antipathy or annoyance. A child's life is at stake, and they both know it. The clinical exchange that they are about to enter is one episode in a much larger narrative that began years earlier. Ronetta has been in and out of the hospital for years, including a number of monthlong stays. She is well known to the sickle-cell and rehabilitation teams. Her father has been asked to attend therapy sessions so that he can learn the therapy home programs he is expected to carry out with his daughter on a regular basis. From the rehabilitation team's perspective, these therapy exercises are crucial. They will help prevent contractures, which have been a special problem for Ronetta in the past. Preventing contractures has been an issue for the whole team, who have witnessed her repeated admissions. Because of her previous stroke she is confined to a wheelchair, and a primary goal for rehabilitation is that she be able to walk again. This desire is powerfully voiced by the child, her father, and the clinical staff who treat her.

In the last chapter, I explored how culturally ready-made narratives provide parents and clinicians ways to "read" (and often "misread") the minds of one another. I tried to show how misreadings are furthered through subsequent familiar stranger stories that circulate among patients and staff, helping to reinforce us/them divides. Here I consider how this same prefiguring influences the active shaping of a lived story—the narrative construction of the encounter itself. In chapter 2 I argued that we narratively prefigure experiences we have not yet had. I return to the notion of prefiguring as an aspect of our historical consciousness, integral to experience. Experience and understanding are inevitably intertwined with our historical inheritance, one that prepares us to experience in a particular way. Our historical consciousness is thus a practical consciousness, orienting us to our everyday situations in which we are required to take action. Because we are, above all, practical beings, immersed in the activities of everyday life, this historical consciousness is primarily directed, not to the past or to passive understanding, but to action, which is necessarily oriented to the future. As actors, we enter each circumstance armed with foreknowing, as Heidegger puts it. We prefigure and prejudge what we encounter, Gadamer announces, and this is necessary to knowing anything at all. Traditions, which we inherit, give us our preconceptions upon which our understandings of others and of our situations are based (Thompson 1984). We necessarily prejudge, and this prejudice is what we inevitably bring to any situation.

Because we approach each present with an "embodied history" that preunderstands, we are prepared to misunderstand, to not recognize or attend to features of any current situation that mismatch the (historically informed and tacit) expectations brought to it. All social encounters involve anticipating of this sort. We project before ourselves the meaning of the "whole," a kind of temporal meaning-shape that gives us specific expectations of what others will do, what they are thinking, and what is likely to happen next. We come to any situation armed with cultural resources that equip us with the capacity to "foreknow" what will occur. "This recognition that all understanding inevitably involves some prejudice gives the hermeneutical problem its real thrust" (Gadamer 2004:272). Practical life is fraught with both mystery and hermeneutic trouble. We will always misunderstand, in this hermeneutic sense, because of the temporal structure of understanding itself, which relies upon anticipation of what will happen and what we will experience: an anticipatory story.

The genres of healing I outlined in chapter 2 provide an essential background to the preunderstandings that patients, families, and clinicians bring to their encounters. These genres provide the cultural frames that allow participants to anticipate how events will unfold. In large and small ways, every practical circumstance (and some more than others), because of its historical particularity, will diverge from culturally shaped expectations. There will always be some gap between any anticipated whole and what actually unfolds. If, as Aristotle argues, we always act in circumstances that are in certain respects necessarily unique, then it follows that our apprehensions and sense-making categories, our prejudgments, offer a basis for understanding that is also inevitably a misunderstanding. There can be no understanding without misunderstanding, as Friedrich Schleiermacher (1998), writing in the early 1800s, famously said. This ongoing confrontation with *misunderstanding* is an essential aspect of practical know-how.[1]

In what follows I will describe the encounter that unfolds between Marcia and Ron to consider not only the narrative prefiguring that they act upon (and therefore enact) in their interactions but also the tragedy of the encounter. From the poststructuralist practice perspectives exemplified by Foucault and Bourdieu, this tragedy is already explained by the social institutions themselves: their gestures, their spaces, their economics, the pastoral reasoning of their experts, and the already given dispositions that participants bring to their interaction. From such perspectives, the history of clinical care and its governmentalities, as well as the history of race, class, and inequality in America, makes this encounter a foregone conclusion.

But I want to treat the encounter from a dramatistic perspective that opens up the possibility of action. From this perspective, the conflict that ensues between therapist and father *could have been otherwise.* The foreknowing, the "already there" prejudgment of practical life (part of what Bourdieu might call the "habitus") is not the sum total of meaning making. Rather, it is only the start. The historical givenness of life is not an ending point but serves as the *beginning* of understanding. It can also happen that everyday life brings with it situations where this preunderstanding seems inadequate or somehow wrong. Misunderstanding carries with it the potential for a critical reexamination of the horizon one brought to the situation and the expectations it generated.[2] Sometimes understanding involves an encounter that leads to personal and even social change. Unexpectedness can engender a process of reimagining past, present, and future. This can mean anything from small revisions in perspective to a wholesale reenvisioning of frameworks for living. The present may offer the possibility of an encounter that challenges previous expectations and brings about a "widening of horizons."

If the conflict between Marica and Ron is not a foregone conclusion, then we open an analytic space to puzzle about why and how this encounter unfolds in such a way that the participants' expectations are *not* interrupted. It is true that we come to each situation aided (and burdened) by resources that confirm our point of view and that seduce us into having experiences that seem only to reaffirm our initial apprehensions and expectations. But actors are not necessarily destined to live out these prefigured stories.

As we shall see, not only are the misunderstanding and misapprehensions with which Marcia and Ron enter the sessions confirmed, but the gap between them widens. No critical reexamination occurs. Yet neither Marcia nor Ron wishes this to be so. Neither wants a fight. Both are worried and frightened by Ronetta's deteriorating physical and emotional state. Both would like nothing more than the cooperation of the other in tackling this. However, they do define the basic source of the problem differently. Marcia would like Ron to change, especially in his attitude toward therapy. Ron would like Marcia to change, especially in her attitude toward him. Each makes aborted attempts to interrupt the "clash" that only worsens as the session unfolds. Neither appears to recognize the efforts of the other in seeking cooperation or creating a partnership. Their actions merely reinforce one another's experience of being treated as a familiar stranger.

THE FAMILY TRAINING SESSION

The small hospital room is quiet now. Rena and Ron are gone. Ronetta lies in her bed with the bedpan tucked under her left arm and her dark braids spread out on the pillow. She waits in silence, tears running down her face unheeded. She looks toward the door. And then her father returns, just behind Marcia. The training session is ready to begin.

Marcia is terse from the very start. She briskly begins by handing Ron one of the splints that Ronetta is supposed to wear at scheduled periods throughout the day. In fact, these splints are full-leg casts that have been cut in half lengthwise. Ronetta hates them. Ron works to put on one splint while Marcia puts on the other. Ronetta, who still feels nauseous, lies in bed as they work over her, wretched and silent.

Once the splints are in place, Marcia moves on to the next task for the session, making sure Ron knows when Ronetta is to wear them once she is discharged home. Marcia reads from a schedule on the wall beside Ronetta's bed. This is posted for the various aides responsible for the splints while Ronetta is in the hospital, but it is also used to instruct family members about home care. She turns to Ron when she has finished reading. "So when are the splints supposed to be on?" she asks, in the manner of the repressively annoyed teacher who has surprised her class with a pop quiz. Ron attempts an answer. He gets some of the answers right but others wrong. She corrects his mistakes, her expression stony.

When the quiz is over and his mediocre performance is publicized through Marcia's increasingly condescending corrections, she moves on to her next educational task, making sure that Ron understands the importance of the splint-wearing schedule. She admonishes: "Ronetta needs to wear these at these times so she doesn't get all bent up like when she came in." Ron says nothing, listening numbly as befits his position as the uninspired student. Ronetta watches each of them, her face screwing up with worry, for she can see that things are not going well.

Now it is time for more "hands-on" instruction. Marcia shows Ron how to properly secure the Velcro fasteners that are used to strap on the splints. Ron tries to follow her lead but fumbles a bit in his attempt to secure them, at which point Marcia takes over, tightening them. It is then that Ronetta steps in. In a soft voice that she directs to her father, she quietly corrects Marcia, advising Ron that the straps need to be tighter still. Marcia ignores this exchange and moves on, showing Ron how to make a figure eight around the ankles. He watches her closely, and when he tries this himself he performs it flawlessly. Marcia makes no comment. Instead, she tells Ron how he can ascertain whether the splints are placed on Ronetta in the correct position. Revealing that Ronetta's earlier correction of her was not missed, Marcia remarks: "Ronetta can tell you when they are on right." She adds, "You can also look at where the cutout is for the knees." Ron says nothing, his expression dazed. Marcia, with some asperity, shows him how to check their positioning.

They are interrupted by the arrival of Ronetta's cousin, Elron, who walks into the room. Ron, suddenly gracious, introduces Elron to everyone but asks him to return to the waiting room while they carry out the training session. Ron adds to Marcia, "I need to step out for a minute and use the restroom. I'll be right back." Marcia, who does not indicate she has heard him, continues undeterred: "I just want to see if these fit," she announces while struggling to put a pair of jeans on Ronetta over the splints. But she seems to be only talking to herself as Ron leaves for the bathroom. Marcia concentrates on her task with the jeans, instructing Ronetta to roll to one side so she can pull them up. Ronetta begins to whimper, moaning softly that she can't move because her stomach hurts too much. Then, more loudly, she cries out plaintively, "I want my mommy." Marcia ignores her, working alone to tug up the difficult jeans over the wide splints.

Ron returns to the room a few minutes later, moving more energetically, less resigned somehow. The following dialogue ensues. I quote it here in some detail, for it reveals a kind of dance initiated by each person's solicitations to bring the others into their "story" of how the session ought to proceed. This dance has its small moments of connection, but these are fleeting and they easily falter. As connections fail, the therapist and father assume increasingly embattled positions.

> Marcia: *(speaking to Ronetta and not looking at Ron)* If these don't fit, Dad's going to have to buy some baggy sweats.
>
> Ron: *(in a helpful tone)* Do you want me to get another pair? These are one size too big, but I can get them bigger. Maybe some bell-bottoms? [a popular style at the time]
>
> Marcia: Hopefully we won't need the splints if she gets stronger.

Ron tries to solve the problem Marcia identifies (pants are too small) by offering a fashionable solution—bell-bottoms instead of baggy sweats. His suggestion attends to the concerns a twelve-year-old girl might have. Marcia responds by telling him, in effect, that none of this problem solving would even be needed if he were carrying out exercises properly at home. Marcia's message underscores that if Ronetta were exercising as she ought to be, *then* there would be no contractures and *consequently* no need for the painful splints. As they speak, Marcia and Ron are working together; Ron has taken one leg, Marcia the other, and they manage to get Ronetta's jeans on. Marcia reiterates her message.

> Marcia: Ronetta really won't need splints if she does her exercises and gets stronger.

Ron makes no reply to this. Instead, he sees a Post-it note on the bed and reads it, puzzled.

> Marcia: That's the list of exercises I need to go over with you today. *(she launches in directly to Ron)* Okay. Let's pretend it's in the morning. Take these [the jeans] off, and then we'll do her exercises.
>
> Ron: Which exercises?
>
> Marcia: *(with real irritation)* Remember? What exercise would you do if her knees were straight all night?

Ron regards her silently, again the dazed student. Ronetta looks worried and whispers to her father.

Ronetta: I bend my knees.

Marcia: Shh. I wanted your father to answer. *(looking at Ron)* If her knees were straight all night, we need to bend them. Same with the ankle. It's not hard. That's all you need to think about.

Marcia demonstrates to Ron how to do various prescribed leg exercises and stretches. Ron acts particularly reluctant to do the stretching. He looks at his watch from time to time. He yawns. However, as Marcia grimly persists, Ron begins to imitate her. Silently, they each exercise the leg closest to them—a brief choreographed moment of harmony.

Having determined that they are ready to move on, Marcia directs her attention to Ronetta. It is here that whatever minimal cooperation Ron and Marcia had been capable of in earlier moments finally falls apart.

Marcia: Ronetta can do these exercises herself. She does them in group. Ronetta, I want you to do some now.

Ronetta: (moaning) Oh oh oh.

Ron strokes her forehead to comfort her. He covers her bare legs and her underwear, which were exposed during her stretching.

Ronetta: (leaning into her father's touches) Dad, can you spend an extra hour with me?

Marcia: (speaking over them) The next exercise . . .

Ron: (interrupting Marcia) I have to leave here by 3:00. *(turning to Ronetta)* But I'll stay here with you tomorrow night. *(then to Marcia)* The social worker told me she wanted me to stay overnight Saturday night.

Marcia: (surprised) She's not going on pass?

Ron: They're not letting her.

Marcia: (admonishingly) Because she's not stable.

Ron: (turning back to Ronetta) But I won't be here until 6:00 p.m. tomorrow.

Marcia: (speaking over Ron) The exercises . . .

Ron: (speaking over Marcia to Ronetta) I just can't make it before 6:00, but I'll be here then.

Marcia: (voice louder) You can do her exercises on the bed if she's laying down.

In this exchange, an important transformation has occurred. Ron has abandoned his role as poor student and taken on one of loving, if beleaguered, father. In his gesture of covering his daughter's legs,

Ronetta is transformed from a body in need of repair to a young girl whose modesty is to be protected. His daughter has also abandoned her role as patient by directly appealing to her father to spend more time with her. A shift from clinical drama to family drama has also been instigated by Ronetta's protesting cries at the pain of therapy and Ron's comforting response. Marcia ignores this recasting of therapy time into family time, steadfast in her attempts to prevent an abandonment of the "repair story." And at her insistence Ron reluctantly turns his attention back to Marcia. She then shows him the soft braces for day use and the special shoes Ronetta is to wear. She is clearly prepared to continue with her instructions, but as Ronetta cries and moans more loudly, Ron is no longer willing to cooperate. In the final moments of the session he takes charge and puts an end to it.

> Ron: *(firmly)* Maybe we should wait and do this another time. Ronetta isn't feeling well.
>
> Marcia: *(protesting)* We just need to cover a few more things.
>
> Ronetta: *(crying out)* Nooo! Nooo! I *can't* do this. *(she rocks back and forth)* Please! Dad, I don't want to *be* here anymore. I *told* you what I want.
>
> Marcia: *(defeated, turns to Ron)* Do you want me to just leave?
>
> Ron: *(nodding)* Yeah, I think she's through with therapy for the day.

Marcia gathers up her equipment, preparing to depart. Ron turns back to Ronetta. He leans in toward her.

> Ron: Ronetta, you can't keep talking like that. Talking about dying . . . You need to work hard and concentrate on getting better. The more you focus on your pain, the worse you do.
>
> Ronetta: *(despairingly)* I can't . . . Dad, can you stay a little longer?
>
> Ron: *(sighing)* Okay, I can stay an extra thirty minutes, I guess.

Marcia leaves the room. Ronetta continues to whimper, arms crossed tightly in front of her as if she were hugging herself.

THE CLINICAL ENCOUNTER AS ACTED NARRATIVE

How and why does this drama of failure unfold with such apparent inevitability? How do the problematic prefigurings each character brings to the session play out so inexplicably, so that fundamental misunderstandings are reinforced? In this session Marcia finds further evidence that Ron is not a sufficiently caring and involved father. Ron finds further evidence that the clinical staff refuse to see his side of the picture or the dilemmas that they are imposing upon him.

While one could speak of this as an interpersonal misunderstanding, it is much more importantly one created by a clash of healing genres. The conflict drama that develops in the session is a manifestation of a structural conflict. To consider this in more detail and to examine how this conflict is produced *dramatically*, I turn to the idea of acted narratives. This session is one more tense episode in an unfolding and highly consequential border conflict, an interaction marked by many dramatic features. It is charged. Things are at stake. There are desires thwarted, plots and counterplots, struggles, enemies and occasional allies. This is a drama that produces personal vulnerability, where each feels threatened by the actions and desires of the other. To consider how this conflict drama is emplotted, I particularly attend to narrative form and the features we associate with it: *desire, trouble, suspense,* and *transformation.*

Mobilizing Healing Genres and Their Desires

Marcia, Ron, and Ronetta all express desires for certain things to occur in their time together and try to thwart other possible events they deem unfavorable. They try to enact some stories and avoid others. These immediate desires can be understood as expressions of culturally shaped hopes.

Marcia personifies an institutionally expressed desire embedded in a recovery narrative of bodily repair. But this genre assumes a more complex cast as it is mobilized by rehabilitation therapists. Unlike the good mechanic—or good surgeon—who can fix the broken part, here "fixing" involves a challenging interpersonal process. The "repair" story, so dramatically exemplified by the surgeon performing in his operating "theater," is embedded within a much less dramatic and often difficult narrative of rehabilitation carried out primarily by various rehabilitation therapists. It involves a very different and far less acknowledged drama in which "repairs" are not the product of a miraculous medical intervention on an anesthetized patient but instead the hoped-for consequence of endless hours of painful physical and occupational therapies. Rehabilitation therapists like Marcia must work *with* the patient and family caregivers as well. Repair necessarily depends upon the cooperation of these crucial others. Thus the clinical desire to repair a body is joined by desires not acknowledged in the authorized plot. Clinical hope here depends not only on clinical expertise in performing therapeutic exercises with patients but on the more difficult skill of turning those tasks over to patients and families themselves. Because of the chronicity of Ronetta's illness, the staff's desire is not for "cure" but for the kind of measurable progress that means Ronetta can be successfully discharged and sent home. It is this hopeful drama they attempt to enact. Narrative expectations like Marcia's about how things *should* unfold are also organized materially through, for example, charts posted on Ronetta's hospital room wall that explain how and when home exercise programs are to be carried out and that Ron is to read aloud.

The clinical staff's quite explicit focus on repair is not the only one at play. They also implicitly invoke a healing genre of personal transformation. But they envision this as manifested in the family's increased compliance with their "repair" goals. If only, staff suggest, this father and daughter would take on the task of these home exercises, a whole new life could result. A nurse who has known Ronetta for years poignantly speaks of her hope that Ronetta will "get better" and that she will "see her growing." This nurse relays a dream she had where Ronetta was "walking and running and playing." The nurse continues painfully:

> She's got to feel connected in some way . . . She's got to feel like she's a part of something so that she can excel, so that she can find her talents, discover her talents and come to appreciate herself.

Speaking personally but also for the staff generally, Marcia also expresses a hope that Ronetta's life will change. She "wants her to have something in her life that's related to her, that's . . . stable." Repair of a body is connected to repair of a life.

Ron's desires most clearly reflect the primacy of the transformative journey. For him, this goes beyond "repair." It is Ron who most directly expresses the hope that his daughter will somehow overcome her pain and see herself differently. This is not surprising because for him restoration of the body is secondary to this task of self-transformation. Other matters, like physical improvement, will be possible only if Ronetta changes, grows more confident, and looks "beyond the pain." From his perspective, an emotional and even moral transformation is the central healing task. Ron says,

It makes me feel sad, really sad . . . It, it stops me in my tracks, man. It makes me wonder, What is it that I can do to better the situation? What, what can I do or tell her, for example, to build her self-esteem and to get her to balance her emotions on a level to where she's looking beyond the pain?

Ron also recognizes that he has a task of changing himself and his whole family life in order to care for this very sick little girl. He must try to create a home for her that fundamentally alters the nature of his current family. This places new demands on him, which he must find the strength to carry out. He must come to know his daughter, be a father who is "really there for her" (as he was not when she lived with her mother). He must find a way to make her feel loved, but not in the same way that Ronetta's mother has loved her, which he (and hospital staff) regard as highly problematic.

Ron thus views his daughter's illness and healing not only as a somatic drama of recovery but also as embedded within a personal and family drama. Furthermore, he believes that Ronetta has her own pilgrimage, faces her own tasks of becoming a different sort of sick girl, something he believes he must try to guide her through. He worries that Ronetta wants only to be a little child and sit on her mother's lap instead of facing the fact that at twelve she is turning into a "young lady" who needs to become more independent and more responsible for taking care of herself. Most important, though, is Ron's fear that Ronetta doesn't want to live at all. What can he do in the face of a daughter who is becoming suicidal? What kind of love and care can he show that will make a difference? Is he capable of giving her enough? Will she always want too much or more than he can give? These are the questions that most haunt him.

Preunderstanding as a Source of Trouble

Acted stories may be set in motion by desires, but they attain their dramatic status because of the presence of trouble. Where are the obstacles here? Trouble so predominates that it overwhelms all else. While Marcia and Ron express intense desires for Ronetta's improvement in numerous separate interviews, the session itself seems to proceed with a marked absence of desire by either. Instead, there is discord from the beginning. Perhaps the first thing to note is the sharpness and intransigence of the conflict that plays out. Discussion between Marcia and Ron is terse, veering dangerously on the outright acrimonious. Marcia, while apparently struggling to solicit some type of partnership with Ron, seems almost remarkably obtuse in her futile efforts to draw him into the work. Her tone is critical, condescending, at times even outright sarcastic. Her strategies for recruiting him are primarily punitive. On his side, he acts detached, distracted, and restless. His daughter, who lies on the bed between them and cries so piteously, serves as, quite literally, a border terrain. If Ronetta and her precarious medical state is the common ground that brings clinician and parent together, she is also a border that divides them. They literally circle her. She is the territory over which they each feel responsibility and even, in some sense, ownership. Whose is she? Who has the rights over her life and her well-being?

In this clinical encounter Ronetta is also a culture broker, though a largely unsuccessful one, who repeatedly tries to facilitate partnership between Ron and Marcia. She defends her father, supplies the correct answers when he falters, and uses other failed mediating strategies. She is the site of a border skirmish that is unintended and undesired. The aide leaves feeling frustrated and defeated, the session aborted. The father leaves feeling overwhelmed by what is expected of him and tremendously worried about his daughter's depression. Ronetta, who becomes increasingly upset as the session progresses, is left alone, sick and abandoned to the endless hospital routines she hates.

It is not merely that father and aide threaten one another. In a way, even the child is threatening to them. Not only is she the border zone upon which they are drawn into reluctant battle, she is also a terrifying common ground, a site of pain and despair. If Marcia seems oblivious to Ronetta's misery in the session, her apparent callousness is belied by her words in a subsequent interview. Marcia offers her own anguished description of Ronetta:

> She gets into this place where you can't reach her or pull her out. She's just like a big hole of screaming.

This graphic image, the "hole of screaming," a kind of living Munch painting, connotes Marcia's palpable fear, horror, and helplessness. To witness such pain and not be able to relieve it is a tremendous threat in itself.

From the very start, Marcia's prejudgments (including her fears) seem to guide her actions so powerfully that she disregards moments when things are going smoothly. In any case, she comments only upon the actions that further her own gloomy picture of a parent unwilling to, as she puts it, "step up to the plate." From the session's beginning, Marcia anticipated that she would not have a cooperative father on her hands. Describing it later, she says, "I think that he has an issue with his wife, his ex-wife. So that sort of set the stage for us, where his mind couldn't comprehend anything I was saying." Notably, even when Ron attempts ameliorative work upon a few occasions, or does in fact comply and follow instructions correctly, Marcia never acknowledges this. She focuses solely upon his failures, even recruiting his daughter to find fault with him.

We might take the caustic quality of Marcia's communications as indicative of her particular personality. But when one looks at the larger institutional landscape, it quickly becomes clear she is embodying and playing out a collective position, one that has come to be shared by the majority of the staff members working with this family. Marcia states, "It's like she [Ronetta] has nothing except the hospital, which will rescue her." This presents an impossible situation from the staff's point of view. Marcia argues, "But I don't think it's a good rescuing because it's not life." She equates Ronetta's pain episodes with family problems, seeing her family as fostering her pain. In the following explanation, she offers a long string of "ifs" that link trips to the hospital for strong pain medications to a family that is not there—especially during the holidays—to Ronetta's never learning to cope with her illness.

> If you come into the hospital every time you have a pain crisis and you get morphine or . . . whatever and you come in—you get sick around the holidays because it's, it's party time, but your family's not there. So you'll never learn to cope. You'll cope and then you'll fall apart. And then you'll cope and then you'll fall apart. So I just see that with her.

While Ron is consistently singled out as a source of trouble by many of the staff, Marcia offers a statement that is uncharacteristically direct, invoking Ron's race and gender to hypothesize why he is so uncooperative: "Is the excuse because he's a black father who's trying, and are we holding him to a lower standard, and is that right?"

One nurse states:

> Sometimes I think her [Ronetta's] father needs somebody to be on his case. I mean, and there have been times when I have pulled him aside and I'm like, "You know what? I am not happy with you. You know, where were you? You're sitting up here and you're presenting one picture, and then you don't show. What do you think it makes these people think? You know, you're trying to hold on to your daughter here. Let's do what we need to

do." She's [Ronetta's] got to feel connected in some way. She can't feel like she's being parked in a wheelchair in front of a television.

Ronetta also sometimes emerges as an enemy, an obstacle to healing, though one abetted by her family. Several of the staff characterized Ronetta's behavior as standing in the way of her recovery. She acts "manipulative" and isn't "doing her part," they say. Many are fearful of a "regression" they see in Ronetta when her parents come around, and they attribute this to the way her parents interact with her. A nurse speculates: "I think she feeds off of what's going on around her, when her parents . . . when their interaction is chaotic she feeds on that, and it causes problems." Another surmises, "I think it's because she doesn't have that consistent caregiving [at home], and she doesn't have a resource except scream and you'll get medicated for pain."

The construction of the family and especially the father as "trouble" is significantly aided through informal storytelling that regularly occurs among clinicians. For example, three of the rehabilitation staff drive to work together, and several mentioned stories they had shared about Ron. This included stories of their own experiences where Ron did not show up for appointments and an even more distressing one where Ron purportedly sold Ronetta's computer. This was particularly upsetting to staff, since Ronetta really liked the computer, according to one staff member who "had spent a lot of time helping to pick it out." Their stories also portrayed a neglectful father who left Ronetta home alone with his two-year-old son. "I would have reported him," one of the clinicians said.

But the staff's greatest indictment is that Ronetta's body is not repairing—there is no progress. There have been many medical reasons for Ronetta's readmissions to the hospital over the years, but notably each time the child has returned, she has—as team members say—been "shaped like a chair." What they mean by this is that it is clear she has not been doing her home therapy program and, instead, has been sitting more or less immobile in her wheelchair. When she returns to the hospital for a new admission, therapists work hard to help her regain her flexibility and strength. The success they have with her in the hospital is short-lived, however. To their consternation when they see her upon the next admission she is at least as constricted as when previously admitted. Thus, from their perspective, they experience themselves in a losing game. Their own efficacy, that is, the sense that they are part of a medical story in which there is improvement and progress, is continually and frustratingly thwarted by the lack of "partnership" on the home front. In this sense, their competence in being able to achieve the outcomes they deem desirable is vulnerable—highly dependent upon what the family does to keep this child moving while at home.

Since repair here requires the support of family, it relies upon a kind of educational drama—training patients and families to carry out certain new routines and painful exercises. This task of education (or "family training sessions") is considered within clinical institutions as a low-status and nonmedical activity, often the purview of therapy aides like Marcia. Thus it is structurally framed in a way that does not recognize its tremendous complexity or importance. The father's position also makes this teaching task especially difficult for the therapy aide. She believes he is demanding what she calls "old-fashioned hospital"— something that therapists continually lament. They often speak of the need for "active" patients rather than those who simply "give us their bodies" passively. This need for the active patient, or in this case, an active patient and family caregiver, is necessary for this educational drama to be effective. But it is not one that the father takes up in any enthusiastic way. Instead, through his nonactions and his failure to learn how to do his therapy homework, he resists the active patient role and tries obliquely to enact a clinical encounter that operates with a stricter division between what clinicians do (clinical work) and what parents do (family work).

Not surprisingly, Ron views the expectations of the clinical staff as a key source of trouble. He shares their clinical hope of bodily repair, but their expectation that he will carry out these exercises at home places him in an untenable position. From his perspective, the exercises Marcia showed him were highly inappropriate for a man to help his daughter do. As a father, he should be guarding his prepubescent daughter's modesty, not invading it by placing his hands high up on her inner thighs, as several stretching exercises required. He felt at a strong disadvantage in trying to raise a daughter without a mother's help:

> I mean it's different raising a boy than raising a girl. Now I don't know if a lot of people understand that, but there's a big difference when you raising a boy. I can deal with a little boy better than I can a little girl. You know. 'Cause I think little girls get more emotional and sensitive about the least . . . the least little thing.

His concern is not only about respecting his daughter's modesty. It is also about protecting his own safety. He is in an especially vulnerable position because he has a prison record. If Ronetta were ever bruised by his touches, he fears he could be accused of child abuse and not only lose his child but face criminal charges.

Thus Ron confronts a serious dilemma. If he competently carries out the exercises as directed by Marcia, he will be trapped because Ronetta will be released home to him and he will be expected to take over this task. If he does them at home without supervision, and if anything happens, there may be trouble. If he *doesn't* do them, his daughter will end up with more and more contractures and may never be able to walk again. A third alternative, an outright refusal to carry them out, will also end in disaster, for that will mean he will lose his daughter to foster care. Worse still, she is terribly depressed—how will she survive if she loses both parents? Thus he comes reluctantly to family training sessions, where he feels subjected to an increasingly acerbic round of "discipline and punish" tactics by the frustrated rehabilitation staff.

As it turns out, the clash of healing genres is subtle here, for both genres are also shared in different ways by therapist, father, and child. However, this shared quality is disguised. As the quotes given earlier suggest, many of the clinical staff imply that if Ronetta and her father were sufficiently committed to a repair narrative, Ronetta's whole life would change for the better. She would be transformed. Contrastively, Ron's worries and fears suggest that he does not see how his daughter will be emotionally capable of doing the exercises so long as she is so depressed. Nor does he see how to assist her without compromising both of them by touching her in ways he deems inappropriate.

The Tragic Production of "Already Realized Ends": When Transformation Is Thwarted

In any gripping narrative, the ending is "in suspense," and in one sense that is certainly the case here. What will happen to Ronetta? Will she "get better" and emotionally "grow," as everyone hopes? Will she continue to "regress"? Will she ever walk again? Beyond that, there is the suspense of what will become of this sad, sick girl. Each clinical exchange has something in it of a possible episode in what is generally regarded—by father and staff alike—as a fearful story. More remote is the possibility of reversal, a hopeful version in which progress will be made, though that possibility grows less and less likely. Key indicators such as medical relapses and readmissions illustrate a lack of medical progress that leads inexorably (from the clinical staff's perspective) to the important question of whether Ronetta will be taken away from her father, trapped in a system of social workers and foster care.

Yet it is also true that this session lacks surprise; at least the key protagonists do not appear surprised by one another. Instead, they seem doomed to another dreary round of exchanges, to repetitive time. The session unfolds with what increasingly feels like a disheartening inevitability. It could well serve as an illustration of Bourdieu's picture of everyday social action as a space of already realized ends; social interactions may be improvised upon in small ways but ultimately reproduce already existing social structures. After all, in dramatic time, some kind of transformation occurs or at least seems possible. This is what makes a drama suspenseful. When desires are strong and there is some chance that they could be realized, even if trouble looms large, participants are willing to take risks. Out of this risky action, transformation may occur and time becomes unpredictable. But in this session no one seems to be risking much. Marcia and Ron fall into familiar embattled positions, playing their defeated roles, even as conflict between them intensifies. There is a small moment of possibility when the father (having briefly escaped to the bathroom) attempts to solicit a partnership, but Marcia steadily ignores him, and he soon relapses into the inattentive student. This clinical encounter is notable for its palpable *lack* of transformation. If little seems to be in suspense, it is because little seems to be possible for any of these actors. If a successful session *opens* possibilities for future transformation, a failed encounter closes them off.

Part of the horror of this kind of conflict drama, from the staff's perspective, is the terrible *lack* of transformation. A stillness underlies the tension and drama of the encounter. Where is the progress upon which every canonical healing drama depends? Instead there is a movement that is ultimately motionless as Ronetta goes from better to worse to better to worse, a disheartening repetition that can even be heard in one of Marcia's many laments about this case. Note the strange tense changes (present to past to present) that she uses in the following passage, as though time itself were confusingly marked:

> When I go home, I thought about her too long and it made me weak. Because it's just like build them up, tear them down. Build them up, tear them down. Build them up, tear them down.

Through an unconscious aesthetic, the therapist's storytelling echoes the same terrible rhythm of the sessions, movements that become routine, building up again and again what will only be torn down again and again. And she moves too, from the first-person perspective of her personal story to a third-person perspective, an opening into the kind of frustrating, despairing rehabilitation cycle that "makes her weak." Ultimately, it is the horror of the cycle itself that becomes the enemy, one she feels hopeless to change. "What's the point?" she asks rhetorically, bitterly. Repeated admissions create a collective dread among clinical staff. They do not want to support a family who keeps returning a child "shaped like a chair," for that is medically risky. On the other hand, bringing in state intervention to put the child (who cries continually for her father) into foster care is also risky. Ronetta will hate them, and who knows how well she will fare medically among strangers. Marcia's actions exemplify an institutional avoidance of vulnerability, a lack of acknowledgment of being caught between two terrible fates.

In the face of this dilemma, Marcia has attempted to impose a standardized routine, a clarity on what is neither routine nor clear. In the session, her risk is seeing too much, getting too muddled, finding herself mired in both Ronetta's physical and emotional suffering or the immense challenges faced by Ron. Marcia insists on having a "normal" family training session with a child who can barely keep from vomiting and after a very difficult and public fight between the child's parents. She offers a common institutional response to an overwhelmingly tough situation. We can see represented in her personal actions a collective response, a kind of organizational denial of the tremendously significant problems this child and her family face. In simplifying and directing individual blame, Marcia can avoid the realization that this narrative is simply untenable—that whatever the "best good" for Ronetta is, it must veer substantially away from a healing genre that focuses primarily upon repair of the body and neglects the emotional complexities of Ronetta and Ron's lives, as well as the social, economic, and other difficulties Ron faces in providing the required home care.

For all this apparent lack of movement (even the child's physical bearing exemplifies immobility), there is a great deal of suspense about the larger drama. Will this child be taken away from her father because he is not doing his "homework" to contribute to the medical narrative? How little is the father doing? the staff ask themselves. What shall be used as evidence against him? Who will have the power to decide, and what shall be used to decide where the child will go to live? There is not a cohesive institutional perspective at play, and there has been energetic debate among clinical staff over this case. Two key players, the social worker and the child's primary physician, do not share the widespread perception of the nursing and rehabilitation staff. While all agree that medically there are problems, these two clinicians do not believe this warrants removing Ronetta from her father's care, and their dissenting voices have provided Ron with some protection.

For Ron, there is the even more profound suspense of how Ronetta will fare emotionally, particularly if she is put into foster care. The "end" of this story cannot be predicted with any certainty, though things look grim. And there is further suspense because this is a medically fragile child, whose precarious state will also dictate what turns this unfolding story will take.

This clinical exchange leads, with apparent inevitability, to an unhappy ending. It enacts the failed emplotment of two dramatic healing genres. Healing as repair of a broken body is the one most present to hospital staff. But healing as transformative journey, though most clearly expressed by the father, is also called upon by the clinicians. While both these healing dramas might support one another, in this particular encounter they conflict. While not, in itself, a highly consequential clinical encounter, this session figures as yet another episode in a highly significant unfolding story in which this father may lose custody of his child, who will then be put into foster care.

Out of this conflict, what is dramatically produced is the mobilization of a dystopia in which healing *becomes* incarceration. This encounter is an exercise in fortress building, in more than one sense. It is almost as though a panopticon were constructed in front of our eyes, an incarcerating stage in which prisoners are guarded and even the guards are under surveillance. Marcia cannot complete the training session—what will she write in the chart? How will that affect the financial reimbursements that are increasingly important in hospital life? What will her superiors think?

But Things Could Be Otherwise

One might presume that, as in an abstract Foucauldian dystopia, surveillance and disciplinary tactics are simply part of the architecture of health care. It may seem that unhappy endings like this one are foregone conclusions, that structural forces necessitate the actions taken and the ensuing misunderstandings and misreadings. How is this moment, this encounter, anything more than a mere example of a historically fashioned governmentality? What does the narrative framework I propose offer at an explanatory level? Why bother to speak of hope at all, one might add?

This misses the complexity and quite specific dramatic process through which something like "family training" can be enacted in such a profoundly dystopic way. From the perspective of Marcia, and clinical staff generally, this family represents an instance of *failed* care.

But this is not inevitable. Even clashing healing narratives need not place the therapist and father in contested positions. In fact, their different underlying concerns about the child and their differing narrative allegiances could promote an alliance between them. After all, the therapist does need a motivated patient. If the father were successful at helping his daughter be more motivated, this would facilitate the repair story that is central for the therapist. Ron agrees with the clinical staff that Ronetta needs home and clinic therapy. If he could somehow signal to the therapist that he does believe these exercises to be important, this might reassure her that he shares her commitment to this particular narrative. Or—and it is not clear whether he could do this successfully—if he could share his concerns more openly with staff, perhaps they could together look at alternatives to having him do exercises that require him to touch his daughter in ways that he finds uncomfortable.

Similarly, if the therapist supported Ron in his efforts to be a loving father to his child, this might facilitate his efforts. And this could, in turn, support the goals of the therapist. Instead, when he does things like pull Ronetta's hospital gown down over her legs to protect her privacy, or offer to get her some fashionable bell-bottoms to wear over her heavy leg braces, Marcia is dismissive. She treats his actions as nuisances, off-topic moments that interrupt the real business of a family training session.

Having witnessed innumerable family training sessions over the years, I know how remarkably different they can be. Although they rely upon an "expert" model and an institutionalized governmentality that is meant to penetrate the patient's body, they may play out dramatically in a way that belies or even challenges this disciplinary framework. When patients, family caregivers, and clinicians cultivate collaborative relationships (as we shall see in subsequent chapters), parents may teach clinicians about how to work with their children. Or parents and clinicians may struggle together about how to take therapy from clinic to home and back again. The disturbing narrative unfolding between Ron and Marcia is not an inexorable necessity. The two chapters that follow reveal how hope may be created despite the structural and institutional barriers that threaten it. In these chapters border crossings *do* happen, multiple healing genres support rather than conflict with one another, and clinical encounters contribute to a transformative sense of hope even when the clinical prognosis is every bit as grim as it is for Ronetta.

In making the claim that the conflict between Marcia and Ron is not a structural necessity, I want to sound a cautionary note and raise some essential concerns. Aren't I adopting yet another version of the blaming attitudes that both Ron and Marcia bring to the session? After all, they think things could be otherwise too. They just happen to believe it is the other person's fault. By insisting on this close phenomenological reading of their encounter, haven't I recuperated and reinforced a stance that blames the victims? After all, none of these actors has much personal power or social status in this institutional setting: a therapy aide is comparatively low in the power structure of a clinic. The father is not from a high-ranking social class, and his daughter, after all, is only twelve years old and is very ill. Even her disease has been highly stigmatized among many clinicians and the general public as a "black disease" that leads to "med-seeking" drug addiction.

Shouldn't we look elsewhere if we are going to locate fault? Why isn't this just an economic problem, a matter of health care equity? If there were more funding for home health aides, one might argue, then neither the father nor the hospital staff would have the burden of doing the home therapy programs with Ronetta. Isn't this more adequately understood as a matter of political economy? Or, why isn't this simply a telling example of how truth and power are so insidiously intertwined in modern bureaucracy that what is ostensibly "care" by experts is actually a form of disciplinary punishment? Doesn't this acrimonious clinical session represent the dangerous production of a "regime of truth" within biomedicine whose claims to scientific expertise exclude considerations of race, class, and power?

My short answer to this is that yes, these structural perspectives are essential to an understanding of what went wrong in this clinical session. We neglect the discursive at our peril. Still, I want to insist, it is equally essential to locate spaces of possibility as they are fostered or thwarted in interpersonal moments like these. These moments not only reveal structure "at work" through the actions of particular people in particular circumstances but also suggest how change of a more overt political kind can develop precisely out of interpersonal encounters. I return to this general argument in the final chapter.

CHAPTER 5

Plotting Hope

I have offered a troubled portrait of contemporary health care and the intransigent and consequential practices of racial "Othering" for African Americans. But I have also suggested that this is only part of the picture, one that easily obscures the creative efforts clinicians and patients can make to connect and build trust across all kinds of race and class divides. Families and clinicians often work hard to develop boundary-crossing skills, such as the ability to "read the minds" of culturally and racially distant others and to "perform" their status as competent and caring. In doing so, they draw upon cultural resources and cultural identifiers that stress what they share. The ability to call upon the small things, a joke remembered, a movie just seen, a favorite recipe, can be extremely powerful in forging bonds. Many markers of shared identity can come into play—we are all mothers here, we are women on unsuccessful diets, we are all worried about how the L.A. Lakers are doing this season. When border crossing succeeds, clinicians and patients come to share, even if only for a moment, a narrative of mutuality and belonging. The ability of professionals and families to recognize, acknowledge, and build upon commonalities that cross race, class, and culture is an important and undertheorized aspect of clinical work.

In examining the narrative structure of conflict dramas, I have tried to show that even an apparently mundane encounter, a "routine" family training session conducted by an aide, has dramatic import

Anthropology's classic investigation of non-Western healing rituals has a great deal to contribute to this line of investigation. Ethnographies drawing upon Victor Turner's social dramas as well as phenomenological investigations of the healing process are of particular relevance here.[1] The sheer *eventfulness* of recovery, so often suppressed in biomedicine, is highlighted in a variety of nonbiomedical healing practices. Because anthropology has such a long and important history of analyzing healing from dramatistic perspectives, this tradition can illuminate healing as a locally situated, socially complex, and embodied narrative act.

Healing rituals across a wide array of cultures have been noted for features that also characterize many clinical healing dramas. These include (1) multiple communicative channels that carry the meaning of events, creating a "fusion of experience"; (2) a rich array of aesthetic, sensuous, and extralinguistic features typical of dramatic interactions; (3) heightened attention to the moment, the sense that something important is at stake; (4) the socially shared nature of experience, which is further intensified through mutual bodily engagement with others; (5) symbolic density, creating images that refer backward and forward in time so that the "patient" and perhaps others as well are located symbolically in history; (6) efficacy linked to potential transformations of an individual patient and sometimes a larger social community as well.[2]

At first glance, biomedicine seems an unlikely spot to discover healing dramas of this sort, and indeed it is important that they are often well hidden from view. Sometimes only the patients seem to be aware of them, or they find themselves in something they view as a drama while the health professional sees it as routine. When clinicians, parents, and children help to engender what Oliver Sacks (1984) calls "births and rebirths," they do so not in mere words but through embodied actions. Words, of course, are likely to play a key part in the action, as they do in any drama, but it is the complex, embodied actions, including nonverbal ones, as these are performed in particular settings that together carry the meaning.

Professionals are often quick to describe dramatic moments in the language of biomedicine so that they appear to be doing professional clinical work, not "playing" or "wasting time," "just being friends" with their patients, or, perhaps most dangerously, going "outside their turf" by directing attention to matters that are supposed to be the province of psychological specialists like social workers, psychiatrists, or clinical psychologists. Sometimes clinicians themselves seem to be unaware when they have helped to create a powerful healing moment, one that speaks to the patient in a deeply personal way. Rehabilitation therapists speak reluctantly, with some embarrassment, of how they tailor their interventions to draw in a patient, sometimes defending themselves (in case they are perceived as not sufficiently scientific or objective) by saying that they need to "motivate" patients to get them to participate in treatment. Certainly the espoused theories of biomedical treatment do not advocate the creation of powerful dramatic moments as necessary to healing.[3] Yet these moments are all the more important for cultivating hope across race and class divides.

I have been considering the children and families who, in one way or another, confront lesions that run all the way to the center of themselves, when bodies (their own or their child's) become sources of pain or humiliation, or when they have cracked to the core. Sacks eventually "recovers" his leg, but for the children and parents I speak of in this book there is never a simple biomedical cure. This inability to return or ever become someone "normal" intensifies the vulnerability of children, families, and healers alike. The impossibility of a simple cure explains a great deal about why conflicts can run so deep in clinical encounters. The vulnerabilities engendered by an afflicted body provide ready fuel for sparking dramas of social Othering.

Contrastively, when clinicians and families are able to create significant expressions of healing together, these speak in quite deep ways to the possibility of hope. Such moments speak to multiple cultural genres of hope and thus help, if only fleetingly, to transcend the differing ways families and clinicians express and understand hope in relation to serious chronic illness.

Families and clinicians not only make differing assessments about what should realistically be hoped for but draw upon contrasting *languages* to consider hope. The clinicians' language of statistical probabilities departs sharply from the spiritual discourses common to many families. It is not that families in our study *reject* the biomedical discourse of probabilities and risks. Rather, they feel it presents only part of the picture. After all, they frequently point out, "The doctor is not God," and ultimately, the fate of their child rests in God's hands and not in any human hands.

Crapanzano tellingly notes that "hope presupposes a metaphysics" (2004:100). What sort of metaphysics? Quoting Crapanzano again: "Hope depends upon some other agency—a god, fate, chance, an other—for its fulfillment. Its evaluation rests on the characterization of that agency. You can do all you can to realize your hopes, but ultimately they depend upon the fates—on someone else" (2004:100). Clinical discourse relies upon a hope pinned not on the gods but on chances that can be calculated by science. Families may accuse clinicians of being too "fatalistic," while clinicians sometimes level the same critique at families who express too much faith in cosmological sources. Such disparate discourses and perspectives foster confrontational stances. I'll just quote a few parents to illustrate what I mean.

Alana's daughter has a life-threatening battle with asthma as well as spina bifida. Alana talks about defying the doctor when her daughter (now twelve) was a baby:

> And then her doctor in ICU said, "She ain't gonna make it till the morning." I said, "I have faith. You watch and see." And she made it . . . I said, "If God wanted to take her, he would have taken her a long time ago."

Daniel and Ella refused to give up on their critically ill infant, who lived most of her eighteen-month life in a neonatal ICU. Daniel said:

> The doctors would say, "Bring the whole family up here. She's going to die. This is her last day." You know, we fed off of that . . . And [then] something told us . . . that baby ain't going nowhere. It's amazing, you know? You listen to them doctors, and then you get scared . . . They tell us all the time that she's gonna die. But we fight. We hang in there with her. We hang in there.

These parents' statements might seem to evince just the sort of attitude clinicians worry about—"denial." Yet such parental declarations represent not a simple clinging to illusion but a very deep and difficult moral stance. The kind of hope they express also sometimes depends, to a rather astonishing degree, upon imaginative play. Here and in the following chapter, I look at hope primarily as an imaginative act in which parents and children, as well as clinicians, are central characters. Here hope involves a kind of daydreaming that takes children and even the adults around them into imaginative landscapes where improbable, foolish, or magical feats are regular occurrences. Healing dramas are often built upon such imaginative acts, crossing not only social borders but borders between the real and the fantastic.

I return to Andrena and Belinda to begin to consider how healing dramas are created in clinical practice and the work they do in border crossing. I examine three healing moments in their unfolding lives. Two of them take place in the clinic. The third occurs at home. Each of these moments is small, in and of itself, but taken together they reveal how powerful border-crossing events can be in supporting the practice of hope. They also underscore how the canonical genres of clinical hope (in this case, genres of battle and of repair) have significance for families when these are connected to home narratives. And home dramas come to take on significance as they speak to and reinforce these canonical clinical narratives.

The first event I will describe is a "routine" clinical visit that Andrena and Belinda have with their oncologist. It becomes an acted narrative imbued with the aesthetic and dramatic qualities that anthropologists commonly attribute to non-Western healing rituals. It seems quite clear, however, that the oncologist in this case is largely unaware of the power and profundity of the actions he takes, ones that shift the clinical visit from a purely "medical" encounter into a healing drama.

In the following exchange, Belinda's oncologist, Dr. Branden, helps to create a healing drama that communicates personal concern and care for Belinda as a special and valuable little girl. This occurs not so much in what he says to Belinda as in the game he initiates, which transforms a fearful moment into a playful one, even an affectionate and loving one, an instant that more closely resembles a "good father" scene than a "good doctor" one. It is only after this brief "good father" drama transpires that Dr. Branden begins his discussion of the latest MRI results and his examination of Belinda. Here he moves into doctor mode, but at the end of the visit he pauses for a brief and neighborly chat with Andrena about their recent holidays. Clinical time, composed of a quick physical examination of Belinda and a discussion of the latest MRI results—the activities recorded in the clinical chart—is thus couched within a family-like time that begins and ends this doctor's visit. The entire clinical encounter is no more than fifteen minutes, but these are fifteen very important minutes. In what follows, I draw from field notes not only to recount this brief exchange but to explore how this clinical time is shaped by doctor, mother, and child into a healing drama and why dramas like this have the healing power they do.

THE "YES I CAN/NO YOU CAN'T" GAME

Andrena and Belinda are taken into one of the treatment rooms, which contains the customary exam table covered with a white sheet and two or three chairs. Belinda hops up on the table with her mother's help while Andrena sits in one of the chairs. Belinda, as usual, pulls the otoscope and ophthalmoscope off the wall and begins playing with them while she and Andrena wait for Dr. Branden. Andrena is tense because she will hear about the results of the last MRI. She waits painfully while trying to be calm for her daughter, fearing what he will tell them. Has the tumor spread? Or, she hardly dares to hope, has it shrunk or even disappeared altogether since the last bout of chemotherapy?

Finally, Dr. Branden enters. He smiles a greeting to Andrena but goes immediately to sit beside Belinda. She instinctively puts her hand over her chest where her port is, fearing that he will give her a shot. She says nothing. He notices her protective move and smiles. "No, no, I don't do shots. That's those other guys down the hall. I'm just going to check you out a little, use my stethoscope. You remember this, don't you?" Belinda visibly relaxes, letting her hand drop to her side.

"Hey," Dr. Branden jokes, noticing the instruments still clutched in her right hand. "You can't have those! Give them back!" He playfully moves to take them from Belinda. She snatches her hand away, grinning. "No! I can have them!" she shouts. "No, you can't!" he says, raising his voice. "Yes I can!" she repeats even more loudly, laughing now. "Okay," he sighs in mock defeat. "I guess I'll just have to listen to your chest." Belinda hugs him and he puts his arm around her.

She leans against him, and he strokes her head and back absently while talking to Andrena about the results from the MRI taken a few days earlier. A moment later he jumps down, telling Belinda that he wants to show her mother the X-ray films. He holds them up to the light as Andrena walks over to him. Together they look at the X-rays as he points out just where the tumor is. He compares it to the last scan. "It's holding stable," he says. "It's not shrinking, but at least it's not growing. This chemo might yet work." Andrena sits down again, relieved of her worst fears.

Dr. Branden returns to Belinda's side, telling her he is just going to check out a few things. He gently prods her, which she now submits to without protest. The room is silent. A few minutes later, he looks up and asks of Belinda and then Andrena, "How was your Thanksgiving?" Andrena replies, "Okay, just my daughter and grandson came over this year. Very small." "Yeah," he says laughing ruefully. "My wife and I planned this big family dinner, and then at the last minute, first my parents couldn't come and then my brother and his family couldn't make it. Then two kids canceled out. So it was just us and a huge table of food. We're still eatin' that turkey!" Andrena and Dr. Branden laugh at this familiar post-Thanksgiving problem as he turns his attention back to Belinda for a goodbye hug. Shortly after, he leaves the room.

The Aesthetics of Everyday Clinical Practice

In what sense is this a healing drama with properties noted earlier, ones that commonly characterize non-Western healing rituals? How does it evince such qualities as a heightened attention to the moment, a multiplicity of sensory channels creating a "fusion of experience," an accentuation of sensuous and aesthetic qualities, a socially shared intensification of experience, symbolic density, and efficacy linked to potential transformations of patient and community? Further, how do its aesthetic features shape it into a performed narrative, with the qualities we associate with a compelling story—drama, suspense, desire, and a plot with a beginning, middle, and end?

In considering the dramatic qualities of this doctor's visit, the important place to begin is to note that for this mother and child every trip to the oncologist is, itself, an event. It may be routine for him, but it is portentous for Andrena and Belinda. There will likely be some news, especially on visits after major tests have been done. The oncologist is privy to secrets about Belinda's body, thanks to exotic tools like MRIs, secrets that Andrena, who knows her child so intimately, cannot guess. This privileged knowledge is not trivial; it concerns life and death. For Belinda too, as for many children, though she may not know exactly what is at stake, doctors are frightening people. The hospital has been a source of great pain for her, a place she generally dreads, especially on days when she receives chemotherapy. It is not a casual place. It demands vigilance. She instinctively places her hand over her port to ward off potential shots when Dr. Branden arrives.

Andrena's heightened attention is directed not simply to Dr. Branden's words but to the whole exchange among the three of them. The nonverbal communication is as important as what he tells Andrena. She too is vigilant, and her vigilance concerns more than the medical news. She simultaneously attends to an equally subtle text, a text she reads in his body and in what clinicians might consider the "informal" or "nonclinical" aspects of his communication. She is assessing whether Dr. Branden is doing all he can medically for her child. Race and class play a key role in the unstated text of their exchange. Will her child, though black and poor, or the child of a single mother, be given good care? Will the doctors try hard to keep her alive? She tries to ascertain this through a number of common means—by trying to get second opinions, by "surfing the Net" to see what she can find out, by talking to other families to see what she can learn from others' experiences at this hospital and with this physician. Although she relies upon all these avenues to assess quality of care, one of the most important means of assessment is the interaction itself. Does this doctor treat her and her daughter with respect? Does he go beyond being a "mere professional," a distant scientist, to engage with her in a personal way? Does he know and like Belinda? Does he indicate that it would matter to him if Belinda died or was not cured? Medical encounters are not places in which such conversations take place in any explicit manner. These are not questions that she—or any of the other families—can put to clinicians and get answers. Rather, her questioning must be indirect, a reading of signs in the clinical encounter itself.

And so, Andrena reads the signs of Dr. Branden's actions. She, in effect, reads his mind, and this mind reading is very much embedded in a narrative she has constructed about who Dr. Branden is and what kind of relationship she has been able to cultivate with him. The power of these messages came through in several subsequent interviews with Andrena. In looking back at how Dr. Branden had treated them, she mentioned that she had heard some negative gossip about him but she didn't believe it. Others had said they thought Dr. Branden was prejudiced against blacks. "I don't know if it's true but I don't care," she told me. "He was good to me. He was good to Belinda. He really took care of her. He liked her. And not just like a doctor to a patient. But like a person, like a, like a," and here Andrena hesitated in her choice of words, "almost like a father to a child."

How was this message communicated to Andrena, that she and her daughter were in good hands, that he would not withhold treatment because of prejudice? This was not communicated in words. There is probably nothing Dr. Branden could have directly said to assuage this fear. Rather, he spoke through his playful manner with Belinda, his fatherly warmth, and his relaxed confessional storytelling about a Thanksgiving fiasco. Such small exchanges hold important meaning. For Andrena, they take on symbolic density. They speak to the possibility of hope and healing. They do so because they seem to indicate a very real sense of partnership with Andrena. His actions seem to say, "We are in this together." His affectionate embrace of her daughter is also evidence that together they hold Belinda's life dear.

Of all actions that Dr. Branden takes, what Andrena remembers best, and what ultimately helps her to believe that he has done his best, is his capacity to play with Belinda. For this is not just any play. His playful ritual with Belinda reveals that he has come to know her well enough to participate in an intimate family game, though he may be quite unaware that he is connecting at such a deep level. In some fashion or another, the "Yes I Can/No You Can't" play is a familiar routine that is enacted by Dr. Branden and Belinda in nearly every visit. It is an echo, in fact, of a game played commonly between mother and child. Andrena often gets Belinda to do things she does not necessarily want to do by telling her that she can't do them. Andrena uses this strategy particularly when she wants Belinda to do therapy exercises or a challenging task that Belinda shies from. Andrena, like a good therapist, will incorporate these exercises into play at home, but it is the "Yes I Can/No You Can't" game that especially motivates Belinda to take on difficult activities. "You can't do that!" Andrena will exclaim, having asked her to climb some stairs or perform some other task that is difficult for a child who has undergone surgery, radiation, and heavy doses of chemotherapy.

"What?" Belinda will respond indignantly, but with a smirk that indicates she recognizes this as a pretend insult. "Yes, I can!" "Oh no you can't," Andrena will reply. "Oh yes I can," Belinda will continue to protest. By this time they are both laughing. And so it will go as Belinda, giggling and mock defiant, climbs the stairs, swings on the swings, or throws the ball to her cousin.

Dr. Branden has mysteriously acquired knowledge of the "Yes I Can/No You Can't" joke and uses it for his own purposes, to put this frightened child at ease, a child who cries and pleads every week when she realizes that her mother is taking her to the hospital again. He teasingly gets her to laugh with him by invoking not just any diversionary routine but one that connects their silliness to an intimate, familial child/adult scene, one that characterizes some of the best moments with her mother. The apparent nonchalance of this play between doctor and child belies its utter seriousness in terms of what it communicates to this mother. Andrena fondly remembers this years later. For her, it offers some of the strongest evidence that she found a doctor who came to care for her daughter as a "little girl, not just another cancer kid," as she put it.

The level of connection is deep in another way. In this hospital setting, where a frightened little girl has no power but must surrender her body week after week for poking and prodding, Dr. Branden not only plays a game as an equal but, in fact, inverts their power relation. Belinda does something that would ordinarily be forbidden—after all, otoscopes and ophthalmoscopes are not the toys of a child, and Belinda clearly knows this. Furthermore, when he (all pretend sternness) forbids it and she tells him no, he concedes. Her no, unlike the many no's Belinda futilely voices on her trips to the hospital, wins the day. In fact, she can say no over and over and over with increasing delight. And, in the end, she keeps her stash of clinical tools clutched tightly in her hands while he moves into his physical examination and converses with her mother. Thus, in the middle of the grimmest scene, comes the possibility of foolishness, of humor, a momentary forgetting of the terrible reasons that bring these three together. Ritual moments are famous for being "times out of time," for moving into emotional and social spaces that transgress ordinary social rules and social expectations. This small bit of play, lasting no more than two or three minutes, fits these characteristics exactly.

Dr. Branden would very likely say that he was just "being pleasant" to Belinda and her mother, or that he was "calming Belinda down," or some other small and modest assessment of his friendly and respectful attitude to mother and child. In interviews, he spoke of the clinical situation with Belinda, which concerned him greatly, but he would never think to recount something so "trivial" as his little "Yes I Can" games with her or his "chitchat" with Andrena about Thanksgiving dinner. Yet it is precisely the embedding of the strictly clinical within a kind of family drama, the three of them together, that carries tremendous weight. He orchestrates an interaction where he and Belinda play while Andrena laughs as appreciative audience. This creates a healing drama, a moment that holds promise even when the medical news is not especially good.

Dr. Branden's storytelling also reinforces the sensuous, embodied messages communicated by the play between doctor and child. Dr. Branden points toward a family scene and crosses professional/patient boundaries when he recounts Thanksgiving mishaps at his house. He and Andrena jokingly exchange knowing glances about the family dramas that are so likely to accompany traditional holidays. Even more important, by referring to a common holiday, one celebrated across gender, race, class, and ethnic barriers, a quintessentially American holiday, he also initiates a common identification. This story says we are not just on opposite sides of every divide, we also all share Thanksgiving moments. This storytelling, so far from biomedical talk, carries the implicit message that we are all people together here. Notably, he has told a confessional Thanksgiving story. He does not triumph in his little tale but is instead the unwitting victim of more powerful family members who fail to show up to dinner as promised. He may be the expert in his role as doctor, but as a family member who cooks too much turkey and has a hard time with his relatives, he seems to share a space with Andrena. Here again, the prevailing power structure of the clinic is quietly and fleetingly overturned. A level playing field, even a homey space, momentarily appears. As with so many ritual moments, we find ourselves in a "time out of time" and in a liminal space.

When Healing Dramas "Pile Up"

Charged clinical moments that engender hope rarely do so because they draw upon a single healing genre. Rather, they are more likely to invoke several at once. In fact, hope and possibility are most apparent when a clinical encounter is an episode in multiple healing dramas. Healing dramas pile up, one on top of the other, creating a density of meaning. The moments of a clinical exchange register as significant acts in several stories all at once.

For both Andrena and Dr. Branden, the primary drama focuses upon a battle against disease. In Andrena's eyes, this small exchange takes its place, and gains its symbolic weight, as an episode in an unfolding story that centers upon the drama of cancer itself. Has the tumor grown and spread? Has it shrunk or disappeared altogether? Is it the same? It is this issue, the few sentences the oncologist utters, gesturing with his hand to offer Andrena a visual image of what he is saying, while they look together at the X-ray films that constitutes the life and death matter of this clinical visit. Here too, in a moment so unlike his play with Belinda, a ritual density arises from the multiple sensual channels in which messages are communicated. Dr Branden speaks as he and Andrena gaze at the shadows on the films.

This is "an experience" for Andrena, and one that, at this moment at least, while both look attentively at the X-ray films, brings her and the doctor together in a shared time of intensity. It is another episode in which she feels that the three of them are in a battle together, comrades in arms, so to speak. Andrena is more than a symbolic soldier in this battle. She administers some of the chemotherapy to her daughter at home. Supplied from the hospital by this chemical weapon, she "attacks" her daughter's cancerous cells. Part of what she is doing is seeing whether her work in the trenches is succeeding. The doctor serves as a kind of general, the behind-the-scenes strategist who develops the battle plan, including deciding just what weapons will be used, where and how to best attack, and when tactics or weapons need to be modified. He also deploys an array of troops, including nurses, radiologists, technicians, and, increasingly, parents themselves.

The doctor is also guide and messenger. He can travel into the very inner recesses of Belinda's body and bring back secret messages that he then deciphers and delivers to Andrena. How important it is to trust a messenger who journeys to such hidden places and who has the power to decode the mysterious texts he returns with. (And how worrisome. After all, Hermes himself was a trickster god, infamous for his unreliable messages.) Here, too, the doctor as detective is invoked. Even when a diagnosis has been made, detective work often continues throughout the course of treatment, especially in medically complex cases. Is the treatment protocol working effectively? Is it creating problematic side effects? In Western biomedicine, since the treatment is often so toxic (chemical warfare is not uncommon), detective work is very often required to discern side effects that may prove pernicious or even fatal. In a battle, there is always the possibility of "friendly fire" and collateral damage as strikes intended for the enemy lead to casualties among those one is trying to protect.

In this encounter, the act of perusing the X-rays together is part of a survey of the current "battlefield" and an enemy body count (how many of those enemy cells have we managed to kill?). It is also the site of what is an ongoing medical mystery, at least for the mother. She too is transformed into a medical detective, or at least "Watson," Holmes's loyal assistant. The X-ray serves as a pivotal sleuthing instrument, a technologically complex permutation of the magnifying glass. With it, not only is the doctor able to gaze into things hidden from the naked eye, but, like an expert detective, he (ideally) knows what he sees. Even though Andrena has access to the same "magnifying glass," she must rely on him to tell her what it reveals, what the meaning of a smudge or shadow is, what clues are revealed about the culprit who lies hidden in the depths of her daughter's body. She is intent on learning what she can as she follows his clinical gaze.

Healing as Transformative Journey

This clinical exchange gives Andrena hope because it offers some relief from her worst fear about the battle against cancer (that she and her doctor/general are losing). Her hope that she is doing all she can for her daughter thus rests upon the possibilities that these two clinical plots invoke: that the enemy cancer will be vanquished and that this doctor will sleuth out clues that allow him to detect the operations of an especially devious criminal disease. In turn, this hope rests upon Andrena's trust that she can rely upon her doctor's detective skills. But *this* trust, as we have seen, rests upon her ability to traverse the clinical border zone. For what she must also trust is that she has been a skilled enough traveler to ensure that her doctor is drawing upon his medical skills as general and as detective for her daughter.

As Andrena lives out the story of her daughter's illness, this small moment, a single routine visit between an oncologist and his patient, also takes on its profound meaning as part of a complex healing drama that involves Andrena's ability to cross this cultural border space successfully. As we already know, this border drama began long before Dr. Branden was on the scene, in the year of Belinda's increasing illness and her fruitless attempts to get an accurate diagnosis from doctors. Suddenly, everything changed with a diagnosis more horrifying than Andrena had imagined possible and with the subsequent plunging of Belinda and her mother into an intense and uncertain journey through the medical world—as her daughter received painful but necessary treatments and as prognoses changed from month to month. In this terrible place, Andrena felt she had come upon a doctor she could trust. Finding a good doctor is a measure of her own goodness and worth as a parent. The moral responsibility she still bears for somehow not managing to get her child diagnosed earlier is palpable. Why did I listen to all those other doctors? she still asks herself. Should I have fought harder? Why was I so compliant when doctors diagnosed Belinda with flu or allergies and recommended changing her diet?

Her own sense that she has done everything possible for her daughter, that she has given Belinda the best possible life despite her illness, hinges significantly on her relationship with Dr. Branden. For if she felt she had allowed her daughter to be treated by someone who would not do everything, who was prejudiced or incompetent, and who therefore denied or was ignorant of experimental medical trials or the latest treatment techniques, how could she live with herself? A best possible life for Belinda is one in which Andrena is assured that she, and those she has allowed to treat her daughter, have done everything they could, have acted not only as professionals but with a kind of personal commitment that will transcend the obstacles of race and class. Even when she later hears that Dr. Branden is prejudiced she does not waver in her opinion that she did the best for her daughter. She prides herself and her daughter for their capacity to break through color barriers, to pull this doctor into a common humanity. Moments such as the "Yes I Can" game or the casual exchange of a Thanksgiving story serve as reassuring indicators that she and her daughter have forged a trustworthy relationship. She does not, in other words, simply have trust in this doctor. Andrena and the clinician *actively* created and cultivated this trust. She trusts her own skills and those of her affectionate daughter to forge bonds of compassion. His playfulness, the gentleness of his hand on Belinda's back as he talks to Andrena, are the signs she reads to assess her own ability to bring this doctor into a genuine connection with her and her child.

Yet none of this provides Andrena a sufficient narrative of hope. These canonical dramatic genres still offer a surface and utopian portrait of healing, especially in a situation as medically precarious as this. Even if the cancer is eventually vanquished, the battle has cost Belinda a great deal. Because of radiation, surgery, and chemotherapy, she has lost a large part of her hearing, she has suffered brain damage, and her balance and fine motor coordination may be permanently impaired.

What does it mean to hope here? From Andrena's perspective, this involves her own transformative journey as she comes to reimagine what a hopeful life, even the best possible life, may be for herself and her child, who may be dying. This clinical encounter evokes hope in a very subtle way. On the one hand, it is an episode within a story in which Belinda is given back her life, where she is gradually cured so that she can grow up like any other little girl. While a stable tumor is not the best news, compared to all the time when the tumor grew unchecked, even its arrest is a sign of life. But this encounter is also a potential moment, a next significant episode in a tragically foreshortened life, one where the meaning of this game or this test result has to do with living as well as possible, fighting as hard as possible, with all the days one has left. The same encounter furthers both plots simultaneously.

In the following clinical encounter, the drama of hope as transformative journey is even more apparent. It is invoked as a complex subjunctive hope during a playful therapeutic exchange between an occupational therapist and Belinda. During this period of Belinda's illness, Andrena and Belinda spent at least two days a week at the hospital; physical and occupational therapy began to play a regular part in their lives. Tuesdays were "chemo." Thursdays were outpatient rehabilitation therapies. For Belinda, Thursdays were the best days, especially since there was a physical therapist Belinda was particularly fond of. Andrena credited this clinician with teaching Belinda to walk again after surgery, a healing drama of momentous proportions when one hopes for a child to recover. Additionally, Belinda loved her therapy days because she did not get a shot and she got a chance to play with some new people who, sometimes at least, knew how to have fun. What follows is an example from a session with a clinician Belinda was very attached to, a talented occupational therapist.

DINOSAUR STEW

Here is the setting: a little room with a small table and child-sized chairs. Belinda is busy heading to all the possible toys of interest. She particularly loves the closets, which might have interesting toys in them. (She sometimes seems to think of therapy time as a trip to a giant toy store.) Andrena and I sit in small child chairs by the door, away from Theresa (the therapist) and Belinda. Theresa finally settles Belinda at the small table, poking into a little box of Theraputty (bright yellow, the consistency of the silly putty I played with as a child) that has some marbles in it. I now turn to ten minutes into this session to recount a transformative moment of therapy time. It might not have the drama of Sacks's Mendelssohn-inspired metamorphosis when his leg "awakens," but in its own way it marks precisely the kind of subjunctive time that speaks to transformative possibilities that go well beyond this session. A very impaired and uncooperative child becomes a delighted, mischievous, socially engaged one. Andrena's Belinda—the daughter she knew before her illness—is temporarily returned to her. This is the stuff of hope.

> *Theresa:* Did you find the marble? Where did it go?

Belinda is pressing her fingers into the putty.

> *Theresa: (in typical therapist sing-song accompaniment)* Smoosh, smoosh, smoosh.
>
> *Belinda: (after getting up and wandering around, she comes back to the table and peers into the box)* Where the marble?

Theresa doesn't say anything but takes Belinda's hand and tries to get her to dig through the putty to find the marble. Belinda soon begins to squirm, looking around the room. Theresa asks her to wash her hands, and Belinda jumps up, moving quickly to the sink at one end of the little room. Theresa trails behind. Belinda happily washes her hands and then begins to wash out a bowl left in the sink.

> *Theresa:* Okay, Belinda, I really want you to use this hand. *(Belinda is neglecting her left hand)* Try some of this soap. You need some soap. Here, let me put some soap on you. *(Theresa helps her so that they are both hand-washing together)* Do you know zippers? Are you good with those?

Belinda continues to wash the bowl she found, not using her left hand and basically ignoring Theresa.

> *Theresa:* I'm going to count to ten and then we'll finish those up, okay? *(Theresa begins to count)*

Belinda speaks but her speech is low and slurred.

> *Theresa:* You are going to have to speak louder. I don't know what you are saying.
>
> *Andrena:* *(whispering to me across the room)* She needs speech therapy. Her speech is going. I can't hardly understand her no more.

Theresa and Belinda move back to the putty.

> *Theresa:* How's this hand been feeling?
>
> *Belinda:* Okay.
>
> *Theresa:* *(prompting Belinda to take out the marble and other objects that have gotten stuck in the putty)* Let's take this stuff out.
>
> *Belinda:* No.
>
> *Theresa:* No? How about let's take half of it out. Do you want to make a cookie?

Theresa produces a cookie cutter and shows Belinda how to make a cookie shape in the Theraputty.

> *Belinda:* Yeah.

Belinda watches Theresa and begins to slow down and focus.

> *Theresa:* There's one cookie!

Theresa takes her cookie and puts it on a "baking pan"—actually the lid of the metal tin the Theraputty is kept in.

> Belinda: *(joyfully)* There's one cookie!
>
> Theresa: Let's try another. *(gives the cutter to Belinda and helps her to press it in the dough)* You have to push and then twist it to come up.

Belinda tries and Theresa helps her, occasionally putting her hand on top of Belinda's to guide her.

> Theresa: Push, push, push! Twist, twist, twist!

Belinda accidentally drops the Theraputty on the floor.

> Theresa: *(singing out cheerfully)* Uh oh uh oh Spaghettio.

Belinda laughs. She cuts another piece with the cutter and puts it in the "baking pan." Delighted, she continues to cut out a few more, placing them carefully in the "pan."

> Theresa: Good job! Look at this. *(Theresa suddenly takes out a small wooden stick, like a little baseball bat, and vigorously begins to flatten one of Belinda's cookies)*
>
> Belinda: *(in horrified fascination)* No! Don't smash the cookie!
>
> Theresa: Yeah, watch this. Here, you try it.

Belinda enthusiastically takes the wooden stick proffered and starts pounding her cookies so that they become flatter and flatter. They make more cookies and immediately smash them.

> Theresa: What happened? *(the cookie won't come off the cutter)* How are we going to get that out?
>
> Belinda: Let's get it out. *(mumbles something about a nasty boy)*
>
> Theresa: A nasty boy? Who's a nasty boy?
>
> Belinda: *(with relish)* Nasty boy.
>
> Theresa: So Belinda, do you have a brother or a sister?
>
> Belinda: Yeah.

Theresa tries to find out more, but Belinda's speech is difficult to understand so she doesn't get far. Several times, Andrena looks as though she is going to interrupt and correct, since Belinda does not have a brother but a nephew her age whom she is very close to. But she doesn't say anything, choosing to let this scene unfold without interference. Andrena leans back, smiling at her daughter's pleasure. I have rarely seen her so relaxed. Theresa keeps her attention focused on Belinda the whole time, not looking toward either of us.

Meanwhile, Theresa and Belinda have been putting their smashed cookies back into the metal box, which has turned into a kind of big stew pot, filled with a mixture of cookie cutters, marbles, and other strange things, all swirled in the Theraputty.

> *Theresa:* Are you going to make dinner?
>
> *Belinda:* Yeah.
>
> *Theresa: (looking thoughtful)* Something with *(pause)* dinosaur in it?

There is now a little plastic dinosaur mixed into the putty, sitting mostly on top. Theresa is still trying to get Belinda to use her left hand.

> *Theresa: (addressing the room at large)* One of the reasons we're doing therapy is to get that hand stronger.

Belinda begins to use her left hand a bit. Theresa finds a scarf and ties it around Belinda's waist. Andrena and I laugh. Belinda stirs her stew vigorously, paying no attention to us.

> *Theresa:* You need an apron when you cook. Are you cooking dinosaur? How are you going to prepare it? Bake it? Or fry it? *(Belinda continues to stir the putty, saying nothing)* What does it taste like?
>
> *Belinda:* It bites.
>
> *Theresa:* But what does it taste like?
>
> *Belinda:* Like an orange.
>
> *Theresa: (puzzled)* Like an orange. Oh.

Theresa tries to show her how to use both hands to push the dinosaur into the putty, as part of cooking it.

> *Belinda: (brushing Theresa away, she suddenly plucks the dinosaur out of the stew, bringing him close to her face)* Okay *(she tells him sternly)*. Now, you eat it.
>
> *Theresa:* Oh, I see. You're baking *for* the dinosaur.

Having finally discerned what Belinda is up to—she wants to cook for the dinosaur rather than eat it—Theresa and Belinda look about for something suitable to put in their stew that a brontosaurus might like. They settle on a plastic lamb.

Theresa: He looks hungry!

Belinda: (nodding thoughtfully) Yeah, he's hungry.

Theresa: (peering at their stew) So, whaddya think?

Belinda: (affirming) He wants to eat it.

How to Make a Dinosaur Stew: The Narrative Emplotment of Hope

As a means of more carefully analyzing this clinical moment's narrative properties, I return to some of the elements of narrative time I identified earlier, especially plot, desire, transformation, trouble, and suspense. As for plot, the interlude just recounted marks a shift from a therapy time the therapist later described as "scattered" to a focused and dramatic moment, narrative time governed by a desire, suspense, drama, and a sense of unity that is created out of the whole. Theraputty becomes cookie dough that becomes stew fit for a hungry dinosaur. Few words are spoken, but this is a story all the same, one imbued with symbolic density, a story that signifies.

While the encounter is beautifully orchestrated by the therapist, she never guesses the depth of its signifying power. Understanding why this therapeutic moment holds power for Belinda and her mother depends upon knowing more about Belinda's life than this therapist does. However, the therapist is fully aware that she and Belinda have effected a transformation in this part of the session. They have managed to shift from time that is scattered, where she cannot get minimal cooperation from Belinda, and where, if she is unlucky and this persists, she may have to force Belinda to perform a set of tasks directed to discrete problems (weakness of her left side and especially her left hand, attention deficits caused either by the original tumor or by brain damage from the surgery). She knows that out of an inauspicious beginning they move into imaginative play where treatment of pathology is embedded within such cooking adventures as smashing cookies and fixing dinner for a brontosaurus. The drama relies upon their ability to move into an ordinary cultural narrative they share—the everyday business of making and eating meals. They bake, they make stews, and they feed others. For this purpose, metal lids of boxes become baking pans, Theraputty turns into cookie dough, and plastic lambs and marbles become tasty ingredients for a good, thick soup.

From a canonical biomedical perspective, this clinical session enacts a repair story. As in the previous chapter, healing within this genre relies upon a highly institutionalized drama of recovery. In Belinda's case, the repair work that is most culturally visible and highly prized has already taken place with the brain surgery that removed as much of her tumor as possible. Surgery this extensive does a lot of damage. For Belinda, this constituted loss of hearing, balance, and strength on her left side, language deficits, and overall cognitive regression. The subsequent repair tasks were left for therapists, family caregivers, and Belinda herself. The clinical "mechanics" consisted of a host of lower-status "technicians," a range of therapists and aides whose task is to engage patients in what is often a long, arduous process of therapy. As we saw in the previous chapter, therapy frequently involves the repetition of exercises that patients very often do not want to do. From the perspective of this repair narrative, the occupational therapist's task in this clinical session is to address Belinda's faltering fine motor coordination and strength as well as her cognitive deficits.

However, from the perspective of healing as transformative journey, this session becomes a place for making dinosaur stew, the temporary creation of a world in which unexpected and interesting guests appear and must be fed. The importance of narrative mind reading in creating a shared, acted story is perhaps nowhere so apparent as when things break down. The therapist misreads Belinda at one point, mistakenly believing that they are in a story in which they will be *eating* dinosaur stew instead of feeding a hungry dinosaur. In hermeneutic terms, she brings a simple prejudgment to the situation that proves to be wrong. What is important here is that the therapist discovers this. Though minute, the therapist's capacity for *surprise* and redirection is essential to the way this session approaches possibilities for transformation rather than closing them off. Healing as transformative journey in the largest sense (remaking lives and worlds) depends upon interactions that have such exquisite moments of openness, where possibility is created. It may not be Mendelssohn. It may only be the "uh oh Spaghettios" song of an old television commercial. But there is music nonetheless.

To follow the delicacy of this passage, I return to it with some care. Belinda corrects the therapist's misreading by refusing to cooperate with her. She refuses to push the plastic dinosaur deeper into the Theraputty (good for hand strengthening as well as for cooking). Instead, she suddenly lifts the dinosaur out of the "stew" and tells him, sternly, "Now *you* eat it." The therapist suddenly realizes her mistake and replies, "Oh I see. You're baking *for* the dinosaur."

In earlier chapters, narrative mind reading was most evident as a *mis*-reading not merely of intentions but of the deeply held desires that brought parents to the clinical encounter in the first place. But in this small exchange we get an exquisite example of the subtle change in which a therapist who initially *mis*-reads a patient's mind (or her motive) is capable of catching her mistake and through a graceful correction, redirecting her own part in the unfolding story. Adjustments like this, though small, can make all the difference. Her alteration not only allows her to reinterpret Belinda's behavior but reframes the story they are in. More important than the happy narrative of a successful session is the way the therapist and child co-create a child who can laugh and insist on her way—as though she were just ordinary, just carefree and unafraid. Even her mother exhales and leans back in her chair.

There are multiple protagonists in this clinical drama I have presented. Each comes with her particular desires. But something more than this fact is at stake when I speak of desire as a key element of an acted story. For desire is also something that can, and often needs to be, socially *created* within the action itself. And, in fact, from the therapist's perspective, this presents a fundamental practical problem. If she cannot create any desire in Belinda to participate in the session, she will not be able to do any exercises with her at all. This is a tricky business because Belinda, in fact, is perfectly content to wander about the therapy room—in fact, she finds too many things of interest as she opens cabinet drawers to see what toys might be found. Theresa's goal is to find a way to channel Belinda's energy into a set of focused tasks that will allow her to work on the designated therapeutic tasks but enfold them into activities that compel Belinda's attention.

Theresa makes a few aborted tries, attempting to get her to search for marbles in a box of Theraputty or to work a zipper, but something like a healing drama begins only when Theresa has the idea of "making cookies." Belinda is interested in this. Theresa further seduces Belinda into a "baking story" by violating the usual cooking rules. She introduces a breach that compels Belinda's full attention when she suddenly takes a wooden stick and begins smashing the "cookies" they have been making. "No!" Belinda protests, utterly enthralled at this unexpected turn of events. "Don't smash the cookie!" At this moment, the "plot" has thickened, and it is clear that this is not an expected cooking session. It is marked not by predictable time (one cookie after another) but by dramatic time, where it is not clear what will happen next.

This point marks a key *transformation* in the session. Transformation, as I have mentioned, is critical to the plot structure of narrative. In this session, a series of transformations or turning points occur, conferring a sense of movement on the activities. It is not simply that scattered time is transformed into an imaginative dinner event in which a dinosaur (evidently a rather uncooperative one) is expected to eat. There is also a more potent transformation. The little girl who initially appears unsocial, even oblivious of others, scattered, difficult to understand—in short, a little girl presenting some clear cognitive deficits—is transformed into a highly social and engaged girl who has the power to shape a plot she cares about. Even the quality of her speech changes— where at first she spoke in a blurry, low voice, now her words become stronger and clearer.

The cultivation of *trouble* marks this therapist's skill at creating a dramatic moment. Even the happy story, the one that ends well, takes us through a drama of plight—a lack or need that sets the story in motion, that propels the protagonist in a quest to obtain his goal through the overcoming of a series of obstacles. In attempting to set a therapeutic story in motion, Theresa introduces trouble in a classic way. Through her "breach" of a cooking ritual, cookie baking suddenly becomes cookie smashing. To Belinda's delight, Theresa herself becomes Trouble, suddenly shifting from responsible adult to bad child, enthusiastically breaking the rules and encouraging Belinda to do the same. This playful Trouble is used to attack the deep Trouble that both are presented with—Belinda is living with a body that is becoming weaker and weaker, despite efforts of clinicians and family to build back her strength. The therapist does not, of course, try to invent this sort of trouble for her patient. It comes with the illness.

The emergent and social character of this little acted story provides suspense. What will one do after smashing cookies? What does one feed a dinosaur after all? But the dramatic qualities of this narrative are not confined to the small surprises that move this plot along. All of the narrative elements I have just reviewed take their deepest dramatic meaning when this clinical session is placed within the unfolding and uncertain drama of Belinda's (and her mother's) unfolding life. The therapist's ability to follow the "pacing" of Belinda and to build opportunistically on what intrigues her allows all of us, as actors or audience, to enter the "same story," to create a healing story for the space of a therapy session. But, as with the session with Dr. Branden, the real drama is revealed only when placed in the context of the larger family dramas. This session connects Belinda to everyday life in the sense that it plays out a familiar childhood scene. Belinda, like other children her age, loves nothing more than playing at being grown-up, and cooking is a quintessential everyday activity reserved for those older than herself. But it derives dramatic potency from the way it disconnects; it creates a breach from the life Belinda has been living since her illness. Theresa and Belinda make an upside-down story of her current life.

This little performed narrative connects clinic life to a hopeful plot Andrena is fiercely trying to live out, despite the devastating losses that have recently occurred. This story is one where Belinda has a joyful childhood, where she lives to the fullest. This hopeful plot requires much nurturing because it runs counter to the life story that has been unfolding. It is an inverse story in light of the many losses of her recent life. Here is a brief catalog of the most important ones: (1) she leaves preschool, which she loves, and stays home all the time away from her friends; (2) her father moves out and her parents are now divorcing; (3) she and her mother move from a small rental house to an apartment because her mother has been fired (missing too many days because of Belinda's illness) and can no longer pay the rent on the house; (4) since they are now cramped for space, her twenty-three-year-old sister who had been living at home moves out, taking her son—who is Belinda's age and is very close to Belinda—along with her; (5) Belinda leaves her old neighborhood and now lives in a place with no yard; (6) Belinda's grandmother is diagnosed with stomach cancer and has become quite ill, and subsequently cannot visit Belinda as much as she once did; and finally (7) Belinda eats so little, has grown so thin from the illness and the chemotherapy, that her mother now gives her a baby bottle because she will eat more that way. Belinda seems to be hurtling backward in developmental time.

Belinda cries sometimes at the loss of school playmates, a father, and a nephew. She is frequently mutinous toward her mother's constant entreaties that she eat. Eating has become something of a battle between the two of them. How much nicer to feed someone else, to be the mommy and boss them around in the process, than have to be the one to eat!

And what about the therapist? Theresa is well attuned to Belinda, but she is not at all aware of how her work fits into the larger life-world of this child. She, and the other therapists who work with Belinda, would be further astonished to discover the way this mother has incorporated their work into home life, recreating the outpatient therapy clinic in her cramped living room by moving out the couch and putting in affordable versions of slides, swings, and child-sized tables perfect for working on "fine motor skills," as they say.

The Journey from Home to Clinic and Back Again

I have pointed toward what is revealed when small moments, single clinical encounters, are placed within the broader dramatic genre of transformative journey. This genre changes the central location of where healing occurs. Clinical moments and clinical actors (doctors, therapists, and the like) are sometimes key protagonists, but they are never the *main* characters. Nor is the body itself, as a site of battle or repair. Rather, the main characters are the sufferers themselves. By this I mean not the identified patient alone but the suffering community that surrounds that patient—those intimate others like parents, siblings, and close friends, who also suffer and whose lives are unutterably altered by the fate of the illness.

I have suggested that when a clinical encounter is dramatic within a transformative genre, this is not merely because of its internal aesthetic structure. Because of its anticipatory nature, how it points forward, a clinical encounter that takes the narrative shape of a healing drama suggests possibilities for a life. Its power and meaning are derived, in significant part, from its position as a short story, an episode within larger life stories that are still unfolding. These broader narrative contexts also bring other key actors into the scene. The session I just described has two key protagonists—a therapist and a child. While a mother is there, she is a shadowy, off-stage figure that sits, quite literally, at the outskirts of the drama. Yet once this clinical drama is nested within Belinda's life story, her mother emerges as a central figure in the narrative, and the primary scene for healing as transformative journey is no longer the hospital but the small apartment where Belinda lives.

To highlight how these two clinical moments I have described in this chapter take on significance as episodes within a larger transformative drama where the family is at center stage, I move from clinic to home. Andrena's one-bedroom apartment is tiny but very cozy. Early in Belinda's illness, it was dominated by a comfortable couch, wall-to-wall carpeting, and a small dining room table just outside the kitchen. With the onset of Belinda's physical and occupational therapy, things began to change. Andrena's small living room started to resemble a miniaturized outpatient pediatric rehabilitation clinic. The couch was pushed to one side, the dining room table was gone altogether. The room was dominated by a ladder, slide, and tunnel setup, which allowed Belinda and visiting family like Andrea's grandson to climb, slide, and crawl.

Witnessing this metamorphosis in the months since Belinda's diagnosis, I realized that Andrena was attempting to recreate the hospital's rehabilitation space. Physical therapists working with children routinely have various kinds of climbing equipment, including ladders and inclines to help retrain balance and walking skills. There was also a large round plastic swimming pool, equivalent to a therapy ball pool. In therapy, this is used for children to jump in. It is a standard piece of equipment. While therapists fill their pool with balls, Andrena had evidently run out of space and was using part of hers for folded laundry.

In what follows, I draw from snippets of a videotape I made of Belinda, Andrena, and Andrena's grandson Roy on Halloween when Belinda was five. Roy, the son of Andrena's much older sister, was six. Since Belinda was too sick to go to any Halloween parties or trick-or-treat, Andrena decided they would have Halloween (complete with costumes) at home. I volunteered to come by with a camera (and some candy) and videotape the kids. I promised a copy of the tape to Andrena. She was delighted. I also brought a friend of mine, Bill, whom Andrena and Belinda knew and liked.

THE HALLOWEEN PARTY

When we get to Andrena's apartment, things are already lively. Belinda is dressed in a white bunny outfit with huge ears and a tail. Only her face shows. Roy is Batman this year, and he, too, is suited up. Bunny and Batman and Andrena are watching a scary movie on television. There are bowls of candy corn on the table. The children whoop and grab as Bill and I present them with treat bags of candy. They each immediately proceed to dump them on the floor to count the goods. Belinda tries to steal some of Roy's candy when he isn't looking. Roy does the same. When they catch each other (which is frequently) they shout protests, half laughingly, half in real annoyance. Periodically, Andrena scolds them both.

While they joke and squabble over their candy, Andrena begins, as she often does, a conversation about food. Andrena and Bill lament that their love of eating tends to make them fat. Both love to cook. Andrena sighs that she struggles to get Belinda to eat these days, but one thing Belinda loves is broccoli.

Bill: (surprised) Broccoli?

Andrena: (smiling fondly) Uh-huh. She loves broccoli.

Bill: I love broccoli.

Andrena: I do too.

Bill: Uh-huh.

Andrena: (leaning into Bill confidentially, one cook to another) Now, I've been fixing my cabbage.

Bill: How do you make it?

Andrena: I just boil it. I mean, I put like turkey meat goes first. Then you add the cabbage.

Andrena demonstrates her preparation, pointing out spices in her kitchen she likes to use, when she notices that Roy has gotten hold of the video camera and looks as though he is about to drop it. She abandons her loving description of a favorite cabbage dish to organize the children.

Andrena: You guys need to climb up on the ladder.

Cheryl: (wrestling the camera back from Roy) Yeah, I agree. I'd love to see that.

There are some other detours and delays, partly due to the fact that Belinda seems very disinclined to head over to her slide. She suddenly sits, almost vacantly, and quietly looks at her candy or stares out into space. Andrena starts a "Yes I Can/No You Can't" game that brings Belinda back into the social world. The game initially irritates Belinda into action and then delights her as she and her mother both begin to laugh at their silly play.

Andrena: I'll bet you can't climb over there, can you?

Roy: (referring to some toy dinosaurs I brought as a present, knowing Belinda's fondness for dinosaurs) Can I look in there and see the dinosaurs?

Belinda: (ignoring Roy and grumpily responding to her mother's protests) Yes.

Cheryl: Oh, yes.

Andrena: (shaking her head) Belinda don't know how to climb.

Belinda looks as if she is ready to get up, though she moves slowly. Andrena adds another incentive.

Andrena: Roy, she's gonna beat you to the climber. Get over there before she beats you, Roy.

Belinda, who cannot bear to lose to Roy, is mobilized. Both children hurry over to the equipment. But when Belinda gets to the bottom of the ladder she stops, looking up at it uncertainly.

Andrena: (laughing) Belinda, you can't climb up on that.

While Belinda still stands there looking bewildered, Roy jumps on the slide, holding the plastic dinosaur in his hand.

Roy: (at the top of the slide, crying out) Look at the dinosaur!

He slides down.

Andrena: Roy, get up there and climb up again before she get up there. She don't even know how.
Belinda: (louder, growing more irritated) Yes, I can.

With that, Belinda climbs up the ladder to the slide. While she is still climbing—with some difficulty because her body is weak—Andrena continues her laughing provocation.

Andrena: No, you can't.
Belinda: (annoyed, and nearly at the top) Yes, I can.
Andrena: No, you can't.
Belinda: Yes, I can!
Andrena: No, you can't.
Belinda: Yes, I can!

Belinda promptly slides down in her bunny suit.

Cheryl: (now laughing along with Andrena) Good psychology, Mom.

While everyone talks at once, Roy slides down the slide twice more. Then losing interest, Roy turns his attention to the dinosaurs.

Roy: (calling out to us) Come see the dinosaur.
Andrena: Come on, Roy. You gonna see the dinosaur forever. Keep climbing.

Belinda gets off the equipment, also ready to quit. But Andrena perseveres.

> *Andrena:* Get up there and climb, Belinda, because you don't know how to slide. Belinda can't slide.
>
> *Belinda:* Yes, I can.
>
> *Andrena:* No, you can't.
>
> *Belinda:* Yes, I can.
>
> *Andrena:* No, you can't.
>
> *Bill:* I want to see Belinda slide.

Belinda climbs up the stairs.

> *Belinda:* Yes, I can.
>
> *Andrena:* She don't even know how to slide.
>
> *Belinda:* Yes, I can.
>
> *Andrena:* No you don't, Belinda.
>
> *Belinda:* Yes, I can, look.

She hesitates at the top of the slide. Then she slides down.

> *Andrena:* Uh-oh, I think she can.
>
> *Bill:* Whoa!
>
> *Cheryl:* Oh, she can slide.
>
> *Belinda: (with gleeful perversity)* No.
>
> *Bill:* You can slide down. Hey, all right!

Belinda, now the undisputed center of attention, slides a few more times. "Look at me," she calls out once from the top before sliding down. The adults applaud. Andrena takes another step.

> *Andrena:* Belinda, you know how to slide? Betcha don't know how to go through that tunnel.
>
> *Belinda:* Yeah. Yes, I do, look.

Roy is standing on top of the equipment.

> *Andrena:* No you don't. Belinda don't know how to go through that tunnel, do you, Belinda?
>
> *Belinda:* Yeah.
>
> *Andrena:* No, you don't.

Belinda: Yes, *(giving Roy a toy dinosaur she has been holding)* hold this for me.

Andrena: Let me see. Belinda's gonna go through that tunnel over there.

Belinda scampers through; her hesitating first steps have vanished. Instead we see the delight of any little girl. Even her bald head, the constant reminder of illness, has vanished, clad as she is in her bunny suit.

I was astonished, later, upon reviewing the videotapes of family moments like this, to see how pervasive this playful game was for Belinda and Andrena. Belinda, who had lost so much of her speech, her body, and her freedom, seemed to find such delight in these yes/no rounds. What was the point of such mock battles? There was of course, Belinda's sheer joy at voicing her contrariness and insisting on her own views, insisting upon a self that existed despite all the "nos" that her world had placed in front of her. There was also a mother's clever strategy for trying to get her daughter to do the "homework" of therapeutic activities outside the clinic. Andrena had mentioned that Roy and some of Belinda's cousins were her "home therapists," and I could see this in action on occasions like this.

But perhaps the most important moral of these small yes/no dramas, from Andrena's perspective at least, was that Belinda did "not give up." At one point, as Belinda tried to climb on top of Bill to get a "ride," Andrena turned to me. "Oh Belinda," she said with a sad smile, "Oh boy, she, okay? She will *not* give up." I nodded. "I know; she's like that." Clinic time takes on a particular meaning when it echoes the kinds of playfulness that characterize family life. But it especially takes on significance when it provides a stage, a common ground for Belinda to enact this resolute side, as the little girl who "will not give up."

PERSONS, EVENTS, AND STRUCTURAL DISCOURSES

In this chapter and the previous one, I have spent an enormous amount of time moving very slowly through what amounts to about an hour of clinical time (when all is told) and an hour or so of family time. In recounting and analyzing such minute slices of interaction, I have drawn upon three kinds of narrative acts: mind reading, storytelling, and the emplotment of action. I have also invoked a discursive level of analysis by drawing upon common healing genres (the detective story, the battle, the repair job, the transformative journey) that provide an infrastructure for these interactions.

By taking such time in describing small events, I have tried to reveal how these discursive genres constitute an infrastructure that is not merely something "in the heads" of the protagonists. The play of these clinical and home moments underscores Bourdieu's contention that culture and social structure are embodied rather than consciously perceived. When Andrena and the clinicians call upon one or more of these narrative genres, this infrastructure manifests itself in their bodies, in the "durable dispositions" (Bourdieu 1977) they bring to the encounter. (Mother, clinician, and sometimes even a child know where to sit, when to speak, and when to listen—how, in short, to comport themselves.) Healing genres are also materially present in the structure of hospital routines, in how the body is examined, "charted," fixed in various clinical discourses and worked upon. In its rehabilitative modes, the repair genre is enacted not only in the bodily techniques clinicians deploy and mobilize but also in the bodily practices mastered by patients and family caregivers at home.

A resolute Foucauldian might ask, What is the point of such minute analyses of particular clinical encounters except to illustrate this discursive level of operation? What is *analytically* added? One way to answer this is to think comparatively about the contrastive nature of the therapy sessions I have described. Take the clinical encounter among Marcia (the physical therapy aide), the father, Ron, and his daughter, Ronetta (from the last chapter) as compared to the clinical encounter (of making "dinosaur stew") between the occupational therapist and Belinda. Each of these clinical sessions attempts to enact an episode in a repair narrative. While the prognosis is not good for either child, clinical hope rests largely on what rehabilitation can accomplish to give back to these children some of the capabilities that their illness (or the treatment itself) has taken away from them. In both cases, the recovery narrative that the clinicians are committed to depends upon an enormous effort by patient and parent. They even take place in the same clinical site. Discursively, we see two largely identical cases.

Partly because these recovery narratives are extremely difficult to enact for either child (they are, after all, so very sick), dystopic dramas created in and through practice have plenty of space to flourish. Both cases are rife with violations of canonical patient behavior that prompt familiar stranger stories that circulate among the rehabilitation staff. Each child has acquired a reputation as an "uncooperative" patient.

Ronetta just won't work hard enough, the rehabilitation staff lament. Similarly, the rehabilitation staff moan that Belinda is bossy and doesn't listen to the clinicians. Both parents are considered to be problematic themselves in promoting their children's uncooperative behavior. The staff complain that Ron doesn't visit enough, which depresses his daughter, and that he refuses to learn the home exercises. Andrena doesn't sit through enough therapy sessions so that they can teach her what to do at home, and she lets her daughter get away with anything, the staff also complain. For both Andrena and Ron, stigmatized Othering and the potential intensification of techniques of disciplining, guarding, and punishing constitute ongoing threats that haunt every clinical encounter.

At the level of event-centered interaction, however, things look very different. And it is the interaction itself that makes a difference. The dystopic drama that is created so powerfully in the family training session—adding another episode to that tragic narrative—is never cultivated in the session with Belinda. In fact, it is interrupted. And not easily, I might add. Belinda is indeed difficult, nearly unreachable, at the beginning of the session. The therapist simply cannot engage her. Andrena, though sitting in a corner of the treatment room, does not interfere. She permits her daughter to wander around the room at will. But this therapist finds the child's rhythm. She gradually brings her into a focused attention. She is attuned enough to be surprised when the child takes their therapy drama in a different direction. And she can act on this revision of prejudgment and help to feed a dinosaur rather than prepare him for dinner. The therapist (like the oncologist in the earlier example) is even able to insert herself into a family joke (that "Yes I Can/No You Can't" game) that helps to bring clinical time and home time into pleasurable synchrony. The fact that this is an unwitting insertion on the therapist's and physician's part attests to the close attention that these clinicians pay to a child, looking to create small spaces of mutuality and relying upon the child's cues to see where these might be possible. In the examples I have given, Belinda's clinicians function as "detectives" but in a different sort of mystery: Who is this child and how can I make a connection?

In asking this question through the course of ongoing action itself, Belinda's therapist Theresa demonstrates a complex form of practical reasoning. One may know ahead of time that one is in a battle against disease, or in the business of repairing an impaired body, but one doesn't know ahead of time that a child will be cringing in the corner hanging onto a bunch of otoscopes for dear life or wandering around the treatment room opening drawers and trying to pull out all the therapy equipment. And even if one could somehow predict the scenes into which the doctor and the therapist enter, how does one respond? What will make a child—not just any child but *this* child—less afraid? Less afraid in *this* situation, given who the therapist is, what she knows about her, what she likely thinks of the therapist and of doctors in general? In her very actions, the therapist assesses a whole range of situational uncertainties. What will make *this* child able to sit still, to slow down and to work with her? What seduction can the therapist create that will lure the child so that she can do her clinically prescribed repair work? How can the therapist embed her techniques of repair within some little drama that captures the child's attention?

Even more subtly, how can she find a way to match her own rhythm to Belinda's (as Theresa put it in a later interview, describing therapy as a kind of "dance") so that they can occupy the same place together? In subsequent interviews with this therapist, she commented upon how challenging Belinda was as a patient because of her medical condition and her general "stubbornness." The clinician would not frame her practical problem into quite these questions, but she conjured images to convey the flow of her encounter with Belinda. Their work together "felt right" when they were in a kind of dance. "I know that's a funny way to put it," she added a little sheepishly. "But I was once a dancer myself, and that's how I think of good therapy with kids. Especially the ones who can't talk much."

These may be very small moments in very large clinical dramas, but they are not small questions. And they are not inconsequential. The practical wisdom that informs these clinicians' actions engages Andrena's trust. At the same time, Andrena emerges as a good mother, for look how clever and delightful her child is being. No dystopic drama is in sight. Andrena even has a few rare moments of pleasure watching her gleeful girl busily stirring her dinosaur stew or laughing with the oncologist, illness temporarily forgotten. We would see none of this if we didn't pay close attention to the specificities of interaction itself, to these on-the-ground dramas that occur in particular historical moments. Practice—rather than being predetermined—opens into a range of possible directions, into a dramatistic scene fraught with uncertainties. It is here, in these small temporal spaces, that the subjunctivity of everyday life appears.

CHAPTER 6

Daydreaming

Captain Hook Gets Speech Therapy

MEDIA DREAMSCAPES AS A LINGUA FRANCA OF HOPE

In a borderland like the hospital, the work of culture emerges as a process of constant innovation based on "borrowing" cultural objects from somewhere else. Perhaps nowhere is this penchant for borrowing so creative as in the infusion of children's popular culture into clinical work. This infusion is sometimes used to profound effect in creating transformative clinical moments that speak to hope. The highly narrative language of children's mass media (films and television shows) especially offers a readily available "lingua franca" for creating not only a sense of common ground but also imaginary spaces and hopeful dreams. In turning to children's popular culture, we will see that the healing genre of the transformative journey can take many shapes. This genre provides, or perhaps even requires, a fertile work of imagination as children and clinicians "indigenize" popular media for their own purposes.

The unexpectedness of this resource is perhaps why I took so long to notice it. Take Pocahontas, for example. The first time I met her in a hospital was in the mid-1990s. Of course as an American I had known her since childhood. But I had forgotten all about her until she appeared, quite unexpectedly, in hospitals in Chicago and Los Angeles where I was carrying out research. She looked very different than I remembered—more grown up, and less, well, historical. She had been dusted

hated. A physical therapy aide who works with children in hydro-therapy talked about his efforts to "take care of the kids" because "half the time they're crying and you're trying to entertain them . . . trying to just get their mind off of what you're eventually going to have to do to them and have them not hate you for it." Another physical therapist commented,

> I think everyone's had the experience of . . . where you go to see a child like the second or third time, and they see your face and they go, "Oh no!" And you're like, "Oh great!" You know? How about a "hi"?

Thus weaving children's popular culture into therapy sessions is a favored strategy for creating alliances and motivating children. Reha-bilitation therapists and aides mention that to treat children effectively they need to watch the same movies that children are seeing, simply in order to be able to understand them. Children repeat phrases or initiate actions in therapy that imitate their favorite film stories. A physical therapist at a pediatric burn unit reflects on the importance of these characters for the children she treats:

> Like my one little girl, Anita, who loves, loves Snow White. I mean it was something. So we would call her Snow White, and we would say, . . . "Let's have you walk like a Princess Snow White, and we'll go over and see if we can drop little things for the little seven dwarfs."

This was such a commonplace aspect of therapy that after several years of doing this research, I simply accepted the regular invocation of children's popular culture as an unremarkable aspect of clinical care. Only during the past several years did it gradually dawn on me how important a role popular culture played in the clinic. I began to see its significance as a resource for creating compelling healing dramas in clinical encounters. While the dramatic genre of healing as a transfor-mative journey may not belong to canonical clinical discourse, it figures as a powerful implicit genre for many clinicians working in rehabilita-tive care. Connections between a child's disability and a loved charac-ter's superability can be used to great advantage.

For example, an occupational therapist came to incorporate Spider-man into her sessions with a child suffering from severe sensorimotor problems.[2] This eight-year-old boy was so afraid of heights that he slept with his mattress on the floor and refused to play on swings, slides, or monkey bars on the playground. As a result, he spent many lonely hours during recess at school and at home while his friends and schoolmates played together. During their first clinic session, the therapist found him extremely shy. After several false starts that yielded only silence, she noticed he was wearing a Spiderman shirt and shoes. She decided that "it was worth a try" to see if Spiderman could be incorporated into therapy to draw him out. When she produced a Spiderman coloring book, "a smile began to creep over his face." Coloring the Spiderman book together was the start of their many Spiderman adventures. As he colored, he told her of Spiderman's great feats and enemies. From this activity onward, a pact was implicitly formed, for in all subsequent sessions "Spiderman played a prominent role." He even donned a special Spiderman vest for therapy time. A key turning point in their therapy work was a moment in one session where he enthusiastically insisted that they go ever higher on the therapy swing (a swing he had once refused to get in), so that even while he was in a "tornado" he could "fight against evil."

The "what if" world that this therapist and child created together allowed the child to do things he otherwise would not have attempted. He became a superhero whose adventures he imaginatively connected to those feats he had to master in therapy time. As this example illustrates, children's popular culture can provide a "key" into the world of a child's imagination, one where the clinician can become an ally rather than an enemy.

A child's beloved character from popular culture can offer a kind of narrative shadow, a cultural resource that children, families, and health care professionals readily turn to in playfully invoking a hopeful future and resisting stigmatized identities. How does the *narrative* quality of this cultural resource assist in this appropriation? I begin an answer by remembering some simple and general features of narrative, ones that tend to hold true across a vast variety of story types and situations of storytelling. Stories put characters into particular circumstances and show us how they respond to and try to shape those circumstances. Three key elements of narratives are illustrated in this simple statement: actions (knit together through a plot), actors (or characters), and circumstances. Stories are about characters as much as about actions. In fact, the connection of agents to action forms an inextricable aspect of the story. Characters confront situations that call for action; they are key shapers of story events, and their responses to what happens are the focal point of narrative attention. Characters reveal *who* they are and the motives they have in and through their action and suffering. Finally, characters and their actions also reveal something about the circumstances they try to shape, for agents never act in a vacuum but always in concrete situations. I have spoken in earlier chapters about how, from a dramatistic perspective (as Burke depicts it), the scenes or circumstances of events can act as agents. The scene can include anything from socially, naturally, and supernaturally shaped conditions to the specific history of actions of other influential agents. Significantly, circumstances are no mere backdrop for actions but play a dramatic role in shaping the outcome of the story (Park 2008). Reciprocally, circumstances in stories also have potential to be acted upon and shaped, for the actions of characters will modify or reproduce circumstances.

As reception and performance theories have emphasized, the *meaning* of a story has everything to do with the circumstances of the *telling*, how and where it is performed, and how it is received and taken up by its various audiences. The central concern here is the connection between the narrative form of media texts and the narrative form of local histories. Electronic media, as Appadurai says, "are resources for experiments with self-making in all sorts of societies, for all sorts of persons. They allow scripts for possible lives to be imbricated with the glamour of film stars and fantastic film plots" (1996:3), and they "provide resources for self-imagining as an everyday social project" (1996:4). The media play a potent role in children's constructions of cultural identities; media stories stimulate imaginative identification and offer models for living (Rapp and Ginsburg 2001). The public stories provided by popular films are quite obviously not models imitated in literal fashion. They furnish characters and events that are not only different from a child's or family's life but fantastic altogether. Their fancifulness is precisely what provides their flexibility for indigenizing as well as their usefulness in creating new senses of possibility. Media-manufactured dreams can offer a cultural resource for countering the waking nightmares that serious illness or disability provokes.

In what follows, I explore three features of media narratives (like Disney films) that make them useful as a lingua franca in the clinic and powerful as a means for contesting stigmatized identities at home. These are (1) their immediate possibility for "indigenizing"; (2) their capacity for creating a common ground that is an imaginary space; and (3) their "subjunctivity," which, as I have suggested, makes them an especially potent resource for the cultural construction of hope.

INDIGENIZING IN THE CLINIC: BUZZ LIGHTYEAR HAS
SURGERY TOO

Commodities produced globally are not passively consumed by their audiences but, as Appadurai argues, creatively made over, "indigenized," as he puts it (1996:32). I offer the following example of creative indigenizing as it occurs in clinical practice. A young boy, Willy, was badly burned on his face and arm when he was just a year and a half old. The paramedics had to be called and he was rushed to the hospital. In addition to a series of surgeries, a major part of treatment involved wearing medical masks. When Willy was taken to the emergency room, he was given a medical mask to be worn twenty-four hours a day for at least a year. His family was told that he would not scar nearly as much if he wore his mask faithfully. Four years later, there have been a series of masks.

The most current version at the time of this analysis is made out of clear plastic, with holes cut out for his eyes, nose, and mouth. Willy has hated them all. Trying to get Willy to wear his mask has been a constant source of struggle in the family. At the same time, the donning of the medical masks marked the start of Willy's identifications with a series of superheroes, a connection initially inspired by an occupational therapist who had made his masks over the years. "Now you look like Batman," she told him with a laugh when she first fitted him. While he began as Batman, over the months he spent time as Superman, Spiderman, and finally Buzz, the superhero who most gripped his imagination.

Buzz Lightyear is a key protagonist in the Disney movies *Toy Story* and *Toy Story II*. In *Toy Story*, Buzz arrives as the newest toy in a boy's collection, a space hero complete with a fancy space uniform, including a space helmet with a visor (also clear plastic) that covers his face. Notably, Buzz refuses to take off his helmet because he is convinced that earth air is toxic. Like Buzz, who keeps his visor on at all times, Willy has been instructed to keep his mask on to protect himself from "toxic" earth air.

Willy's family helped to solidify this identification between Willy and Buzz. Willy owned the original *Toy Story* DVD (as well as *Toy Story II*), and family members repeatedly watched these with him. For many years, Willy's favorite toys included a Buzz Lightyear action figure, *Toy Story* computer games, and, for at least one Halloween, a Buzz Lightyear costume. Buzz gradually infiltrated the entire household, showing up on television, in backyard play, and in games invented by Willy and his cousins, as a masked figure who had come to live with them. Willy enacted Buzz routinely, to the entertainment of household members. His mother and his cousins used to laugh at his insistence upon leaping off the furniture so that he could "fly like Buzz." (Even years later, they still tell fond tales of his antics when he was in his "Buzz phase.")

The adults planned special events featuring Buzz. For instance, when Willy was facing his first surgery at age three, his mother promised to reward him with a special trip to Florida's Disney World. This trip was a major topic of conversation between Willy and his mother. It would be his very first plane trip. Before the surgery, his mother coached him in telling us (the researchers) about it. She asked him whom he was going to see in Disney World. When he replied, "Mickey and Minnie and Duck," his mother prompted, "Well, you know, who else is gonna be there? What about Buzz?"

Buzz "traveled" to the clinic with Willy on his monthly visits to a dauntingly large urban hospital in the heart of Los Angeles. In its own way, the air here was as lethal for Willy as it was for Buzz, for Willy, too, had to keep his visor down. It was not so much earth air that was the problem; it was Willy's mother, who insisted that Willy wear his mask when seeing his doctor and occupational therapist (though she was more lax at home). She knew the pervasive client-professional contract: show cooperation if you want to get care. Wearing the mask was an important performance of patient (and parent) compliance. His mother's insistence made Willy especially irritable, so a visit to the hospital was an occasion for friction and fighting.

A brief description of a single routine visit reveals how Buzz served as cultural mediator between health professionals and family. Willy and Sasha (his mother) arrive promptly for their appointment at the burn clinic, but as usual they have a considerable wait. They are there to see both the occupational therapist who makes Willy's masks and the physicians who will perform the next surgery. As they sit in the waiting room, a doctor who knows Willy well passes down the hall. "To infinity and beyond!" he calls out with a grin as he briskly walks by. Willy and Sasha both laugh, for this is quintessential "Buzz-speak." As a fellow sufferer with Willy (the toxic air problem), Buzz is present during this visit to the therapist not only obliquely but explicitly in a brief appearance when Willy excitedly tells his therapist about an upcoming trip to Disney World where he will see Mickey, Donald Duck, and, as his mother reminds him again, Buzz Lightyear. The therapist congratulates him on this special treat and engages him in a detailed discussion of *Toy Story* and *Toy Story II*. They compare notes on which of the two movies they prefer.

Their cheerful conversation is interrupted by the arrival of the two doctors who will be performing surgery on Willy. Willy is far less happy to see them. As soon they arrive he turns his head away. His mother coaxes, "Look over at Dr. James." Dr. James, in a very direct tone, tells him, "You've got to let me look at you if we're gonna be able to help you." Willy reluctantly turns his face toward the two doctors as they discuss how to do the surgery, speaking in that usual way when clinicians confer, with the patient as a distant third person. "We're going to make a V here and open his mouth some. He definitely needs that," one tells the other. "And we're going to get rid of this pocket," Dr. James continues, pointing to the place where the skin above his upper lip has not grown back together in the center cleft, creating a space. The doctor turns to Willy, "Yeah, you'd like that, wouldn't you? So that you can stuff more food down it, right?" Willy does not reply. Again, there is a sense that Buzz has followed Willy even into this frightening place, for there are events in *Toy Story* that uncannily parallel Willy's experience, including the horrifying scene where Buzz's face is about to be operated on. In *Toy Story I*, Buzz is pursued by a terrible enemy, the sinister boy next door, a kind of psychotic doctor-scientist who, complete with surgical mask and terrifying instruments, tortures his own toys by performing cruel "operations" and surgeries on them. His clinical ministrations result in disabled toys.

Buzz Lightyear's adventures were not merely happenstance parallels to Willy's life. They were reinvented as he was incorporated into Willy's everyday world and traveled with him into the spaces of clinical care. This active indigenizing was very evident when the introduction of Buzz into Willy's life placed Buzz in adventures more terrible than those he had confronted in the movie. While in *Toy Story* the evil boy Syd threatens to perform surgeries on Buzz, he is able to escape this horrifying fate. But in Willy's life, there was no such escape. The *Toy Story* plot was remade in the Willy-Buzz version so that not only did Buzz have to go to the hospital regularly—a place peopled by grown-ups who wore surgical masks and discussed how they intended to slice up his face—but these surgeries actually occurred.

As reception theory points out, the meaning of a media text is not given in the text itself but created within the processes through which it is taken up and consumed by particular interpretive communities in particular historical contexts.[3] Audiences do not merely consume, they "poach" (de Certeau 1984). Modes of consumption are also modes of cultural production.[4] De Certeau notes that critiques of television, journalism, or other mass media generally presume that "the public is moulded by the products imposed on it." This, he states, is based on a misunderstanding of the act of consumption, one where consumption is equated with assimilation and where "'assimilating' necessarily means 'becoming similar to' what one absorbs" (1984:167).

Countering this passive picture, de Certeau offers a radically different view. Rather than *becoming similar to,* consuming can involve *making something similar to* what one is, making it one's own. De Certeau argued that scholars have largely been inattentive to this aspect of consumption, presuming that "the efficiency of production implies the inertia of consumption," producing its own ideology of "consumption-as-a-receptacle" (1984:167). Such inattention has the significant consequence of not recognizing everyday creativity. As de Certeau puts it: "By challenging 'consumption' as it is conceived . . . we may be able to discover creative activity where it has been denied that any exists" (1984:168). Anthropology has actively contributed to an attention to the active consumption of Western popular culture in a variety of communities around the world (Ginsburg, Abu-Lughod, and Larkin 2002).

This "making similar to" and the reinvention of Buzz's adventures in a Willy-Buzz version can be seen in the following exchange between a nurse and Willy's mother when Willy is in the hospital after one of his surgeries. In this encounter, Willy is lying in the hospital bed while his mother sits next to him. The television is on and *Toy Story II* is playing, which Willy is intently watching. On his bed lie both the video case and a two-foot-tall blowup doll of Buzz Lightyear. A nurse enters the room. "I *love* this movie," she tells them. After checking on Willy, she begins a conversation with him. He cannot reply because of his surgery. Nevertheless, he turns his attention to her as she speaks.

> *Nurse:* You are so handsome. Did you wish your mom a Happy Mother's Day yesterday? I bet you did. *(Willy does not respond to this and she pauses, changing tactics)* I like Buzz Lightyear. He is cool. And I heard that you saw Spiderman, and it was very fun. Once you can talk, you have to tell me all about it, okay?
>
> *Sasha:* Buzz went into surgery today.
>
> *Nurse:* What?

Sasha: Buzz went into surgery today.

Nurse: He had surgery, too?! He's like your best friend. He does the same thing as you.

Sasha: He went to surgery and everything.

Nurse: Buzz looks pretty good. *(Sasha and the nurse laugh)* Okay, Willy. I'll see you later, sweet pea. Be a good boy.

The nurse leaves and Willy returns to watching *Toy Story*.

When the nurse walks in the room, the presence of Buzz is palpable. He sits on the bed and speaks from the TV. He is the focus of Willy's attention. The nurse, absorbing this, brings Buzz immediately into her conversation with Willy. She too likes Buzz, she tells Willy, for he is "cool." But the moment of real appropriation is directed by Sasha. It is not simply that Buzz is likable. He, like Willy, "went into surgery today." The nurse is a little slow to follow this creative move. "What?" she asks, and Sasha repeats, "Buzz went into surgery today." The nurse, beginning to catch on, turns to Willy. "He had surgery *too?*" she asks, astonished. Sasha affirms, repeating yet a third time, "He went to surgery and everything," to which the nurse remarks, "Buzz looks pretty good," consummating a moment of ironic play that finally places the two women in the same creative space. They laugh, for indeed Buzz must have had a remarkably successful surgery. He has emerged from it fully recovered, and so quickly.

IMAGINING COMMON GROUND

Such indigenizing paves the way for the creation of common ground in clinical work. Common ground here means much more than sharing a space of understanding. It means the creation of new and even imaginary ground. This construction of an imaginary space is particularly illustrated in the following example, a clinical moment between a child (Gregory), his speech therapist (Naren), and his mother. Together they (primarily the speech therapist and child, but with crucial assistance from the mother) create a common imaginative world by drawing upon and radically revising the Disney movie *Peter Pan*.

First, a few words about Gregory.

Gregory especially loves the antiheroes and villains in children's movies. His favorites are Bruce, the shark from Disney's *Finding Nemo;* Cruella de Vil, from *101 Dalmatians;* the dangerous meat-eating dinosaurs of *Jurassic Park* and Disney's *Dinosaur;* and especially Captain

Hook from Disney's *Peter Pan*. Despite attempts by adults to discourage him, Gregory is reluctant to give up his favorite villains. Instead, he works to bring his therapists into his play world, sometimes even cleverly turning them into assistant bad guys.

Gregory's therapists (he receives both speech and occupational therapy) sometimes worry about his love for these infamous "bad guys" because Gregory, who has been diagnosed with both emotional and autistic-spectrum disorders, is a boy who is continually in trouble at school. He is big for his age (nine at the time of this example). Though extremely friendly, his way of connecting with children is by pushing or hugging fiercely and exuberantly. Many of his classmates are rather afraid of him. He also has substantial speech impediments that make him very difficult to understand, further isolating him. His mother, sighing in frustration, says she would love to home-school him if she could afford to stay home from work. Since he can't sit still, "I'd just follow him around with his lessons," she told us. "He'd do school on the move." His mother relishes his playful imagination, as do his therapists. But they also fear that if he cannot learn to "fit in" at school, as he gets older he will find himself in more serious trouble. Will his teachers and schoolmates see his lovable side, his speech therapist worries? Or will he just be stigmatized? What might be cute in an overly enthusiastic and active nine-year-old boy may begin to look dangerous in a preteen, especially, his mother tells us, an African American boy in a predominantly white school.

What does hoping look like in this case? What would count as hoping—and clinical improvements as a source of hope—from the shared perspective of parent and therapist? For them, it would involve concrete outcomes like Gregory being able to sit in a chair and stay focused on a task without jumping up and down; more diffusely but much more importantly it would make Gregory more able to connect better socially, to not be (the speech therapist's words) a "bull in a china shop." Gregory's mother would like her child to behave well enough in school so that he does not get assigned to a special education classroom.

Notably, in the clinical encounter between Gregory and his speech therapist that I describe below, all these hopeful possibilities are enacted. Gregory's ability to express desire, to make himself understood, to concede, and to entice allows them to create a common space. This is just what he longs to do with his classmates but is unable to. He does so not as Gregory, the boy, but as Gregory–Captain Hook, a hybrid creature who emerges in the course of therapy itself.

HOW GREGORY BECOMES CAPTAIN HOOK AND GOES ON A TREASURE HUNT

I begin where children's therapy sessions often begin, in the waiting room. Naren, the speech therapist, comes out to the lobby to meet Gregory and his mother. Gregory makes an initial bid in the waiting room as Naren comes out to greet him and talk with his mother about how things are going at home and at school. He takes a life jacket from a box of children's toys, puts it on upside down (to create a finlike effect, which he augments with hand gestures), and proceeds to swim menacingly around the waiting room.

There follow a few moments in which Naren takes Gregory into the therapy room (while his mother waits outside) and tries to get him to focus on her. She is very directive and largely unsuccessful. "Look at me, look at me," she repeatedly insists, turning his face toward hers as she tries to get him to talk about school. He offers a confused sentence about a playground game while turning to look out at space. Giving up, she settles them at a small table. She tells Gregory that they are going to make drawings and talk about what they draw. At once he takes his paper and draws a big blue shark, a "meat-eating shark!" he cries out joyfully. He has set the scene. They are in the ocean. Since he has offered an under-the-sea theme, Naren draws gentler creatures on her paper—a starfish, an octopus. As they continue to draw their underwater world, Gregory directs his shark to chase and devour all of her sea animals. Naren grows increasingly uneasy with Gregory's story line and finally says, "Okay, he can eat one more fish and then NO MORE LUNCH!" She heads above water, drawing a sailboat. Perhaps they can go fishing, she suggests. Here is a bit of this snippet in more detail:

> *Naren:* I'm gonna pretend Gregory is fishing in this sailboat. What do you think? Do you want to go fishing?
>
> *Gregory:* (pauses, looking puzzled by this change of scene; but quickly smiling, he dramatically raises his arms, as if he were steering a large boat, and protests, in a cheerfully menacing tone) No, No! It's a *pirate* boat!
>
> *Naren:* (recasting the story once again) Oh, okay. Wait, listen, if you're a pirate, what are you looking for?

Gregory: (ominously and with great delight) For yooouuu!

Naren: No. *(shakes her head)* Look at me. *(tries to direct his gaze to her eyes, a common therapeutic concern with autistic children)* If you're a pirate, what do you look for? *(Gregory looks at Naren, then out the window)*

Gregory: (more tentatively) For uh, for you?

Naren: No. You don't look for me. You look for . . .

She pauses, hoping he will fill in something more socially acceptable. Evidently it is not all right for this pirate to try to capture her. She suggests, "How about treasure?" She wants him to search for more innocuous things, like hidden gold in treasure chests at the bottom of a quiet Crayola blue sea. When she asks Gregory what they should put in the treasure box, he is captivated. The whole tenor of their time together changes—they have entered a common scene that suits them both. They even begin drawing on the same piece of paper.

Ingeniously, Naren also introduces the shark into this new story. But this time Gregory the pirate and his fellow pirates are the ones who are endangered by the shark, for the shark is guarding the treasure. Now there is desire (that treasure) and danger (the shark) and an adventure, the beginning of a new plot. They will be embarking on a voyage to get the buried treasure without being eaten by the shark. After some skirmishing, they move on to the question of what pirates will wear. Gregory tells her that the pirate must have "a big rusty sword." She cannot understand him. "How's that?" He repeats louder, annoyed that she is not catching the reference to the Disney character Captain Hook.

Gregory: A *big* rusty sword.

Naren: A big red sword?

Gregory: No. A big *rusty* sword. A *rusty* sword.

Naren: A restus sword?

Gregory: Yeah.

Naren: I don't know what that is.

Gregory is getting exasperated. He explains impatiently.

Gregory: From Evil Captain Hook.

Naren: Oh, from Evil Captain Hook.

Gregory: (with relish, imitating the movie character's voice and mannerisms) Yeah, Evil Captain Hook!

Naren: Oooh *(in a scared voice)*. Don't mess with Gregory, right?

Gregory: And *you're* a pirate. *(points at Naren)*

Naren: Oooh. Well, can I come on your boat too?

Gregory: Yeah.

Yielding to Gregory's persistence, Naren finally relinquishes her idea of going on a peaceful fishing trip. She does hold out for getting a "nice name" for *herself*, however. The indigenized Gregory–Captain Hook is far less evil than his movie counterpart. He even diplomatically invites his therapist onto his pirate ship. At the therapist's insistence, he is not a terrifying people-hunter, nemesis of Peter Pan, but another adventurous pirate who even has "girl pirates" with "nice names" on his crew. In their adventures, they do nothing more sinister than blow whistles and search for treasure boxes with gold coins and even necklaces (the therapist's idea again). Captain Hook has been significantly domesticated. In the clinic, he is barred from performing any really menacing "evil deeds" such as chasing down the speech therapist. But Gregory resists completely abandoning Hook's sinister character. Thanks to Gregory's growling voices and threatening postures, even the remade Captain Hook is not utterly tamed. Gregory, as the therapist says, is not to be "messed with."

Having finished their story, Gregory practices it, and then in the final scenes of the therapy session he and Naren return to the waiting room to his mother. He is ready to tell her their story. He proceeds to recount the adventures of pirates and sharks and hidden treasures. He even embodies Captain Hook for her in an inspired moment. His mother, the perfect audience, is properly impressed.

This is an especially intriguing example, for the imaginative landscape Gregory and his therapist create involves some tricky and opportunistic inventiveness on both their parts as each resists and attempts to thwart the other. There are struggles over power. Whose story will get to be told? What kind of imaginative universe are they making? Gregory imports meat-eating sharks and human- (Peter Pan) chasing pirates. His therapist tries for a peaceful fishing trip. What they ultimately create is a narrative different from either of these. In doing so, they come to share a hopeful moment where they have created a story of social belonging (they are now pirates together) in a shared adventure. More powerfully, they have *enacted* a narrative of communal adventure, a therapeutic moment of joint experience that delights them both. This is just the sort of cooperative venture that Gregory, his mother, and his therapist dream he will learn to enact in the much harsher "real world" of school and playground time.

SUBJUNCTIVIZING AND THE WORK OF HOPE: CREATING NARRATIVE SYMMETRIES BETWEEN MEDIA STORIES AND "REAL-LIFE" STORIES

One might object that while Hollywood-produced children's fantasies may provide a lingua franca in the clinic, these globally marketed plots and plights cannot speak to the deep problem of cultivating hope because they belong to the realm of illusion.[5] Even those who connect hope to daydreaming are likely at the very outset to draw a sharp distinction between two kinds of dreams. On the one hand, there is an imaginative daydreaming that can open up the world of reality by disclosing its possibilities. On the other hand lies an escapist daydreaming that only sedates and confines us, what Ernst Bloch calls "booty for swindlers" (1986:3). Children's popular culture might seem just such booty, ill equipped to inform possibilities of any genuine sort or to convey the complexities and burdens of hope. For one thing, its stories are infamous for their moralizing happy endings, their "good wins out after all" delusions. In light of the relentless onslaught of trouble most of these families face, how might Hollywood's happy endings offer a vehicle for hope that is not sheer escapism?

To further consider how these forays into children's popular culture can be "provocations," in Bloch's sense, rather than just "enervating escapism," it is helpful to move from clinic to home. I return to the case of Willy and *Toy Story* to consider in more detail the narrative symmetries that families and children cultivate to facilitate this subjunctive work. The happy ending of *Toy Story* enacts the hoped-for ending that will make good on everything Willy and his family have had to endure as part of clinical treatment. This story dramatically embodies their medical hope. In the final scene, Buzz is relaxed, his visor pushed back. He is freed from the burden of the space mask. He has discovered he can breathe earth air after all. This medical hope connects to a social hope. Most important, Buzz has also been freed from his own difference from his fellow toys. In discarding his mask, he takes his place in a toy family, as one among others. In addition to physical hardships, Willy faces the social trauma of difference and isolation. Willy's mother hopes that these medical procedures will result in her son looking just like everyone else one day, that he will be just an "ordinary kid." But this movie suggests a possibility of healing that goes well beyond these hopes based on biomechanical repair. The plot structure of *Toy Story* bears an uncanny resemblance to the events in Willy's family life.

Willy's burn injury was the result of an accident that occurred in the kitchen. Willy was playing on the floor while his ten-year-old cousin Shareen was cooking some food. She was supposed to be keeping an eye on him but didn't see when Willy suddenly reached up and tipped over a pan of burning grease onto his face. His grandmother immediately called 911 while they wrapped him in wet towels and waited for the paramedics. His cousin Shareen was more like an older sister, since both he and his cousins lived in the same household headed by three women, their grandmother, and their two mothers. This riveting family tragedy created a rift between Willy's mother, Sasha, her sister (the mother of Shareen), and her niece. Willy's mother barely spoke to Shareen for months afterward. Shareen was miserable. Willy's mother portrayed her most difficult struggle as an internal transformation from bitterness and anger—including anger toward her niece, her sister, and herself—to one in which she could even consider herself lucky for her smart, young son.

Willy's family has gone through many rifts in the past. His mother and sister are the only two of thirteen children who have stayed close to one another and to their mother. At the time when he was burned, Willy (like Buzz) was the youngest of all the children in the household, and he quickly occupied a special place of favor for his grandmother because he was so quick and smart. Before Willy was born, another child was the designated hero, the one who carried the blessing (and burden) of being the family's "special child." This child, the oldest boy in the family, was a football star in high school. When I first came to know the family in 1997, there was much talk, especially by his grandmother (very much the matriarch), about how he might be recruited by a big football school. (There was even mention of Texas A&M.) Everyone in the family regularly attended his high school games. But in his senior year he got a girlfriend pregnant, and the family dreams of his becoming an athletic star disappeared. When Willy was born, he began to take the place of his cousin as a new rising star on which the family might pin their hopes. When Willy was burned, the family was thrown into tumult and dissension and potentially left, once again, without a male hero.

Toy Story also centers upon family disputes. In the first *Toy Story*, this involves conflicts among a young boy's toys, who have their own secret life when humans aren't around. Trouble brews among the toys when Buzz arrives on the scene. He has a number of space-age capabilities that completely outshine those of the other toys. Buzz himself is unaware that he is just a toy among other toys. He mistakenly believes himself to be a space superhero who has landed on an alien planet (which is actually the boy's bedroom). His arrival poses a special threat to a somewhat dusty-looking cowboy, Woody, who up until this point has been the boy's favorite. One day, in a fit of jealousy, Woody pushes Buzz out the window. Woody is then ejected out the same window by the other toys for his bad behavior. He and Buzz find themselves outside the safety of the bedroom in a dangerous world surrounded by threatening creatures.

The rest of the movie is taken up with the dangerous escapades Woody and Buzz endure, especially their nearly fatal run-ins with Syd, the boy next door, as they try to get back home. Through their trials they become friends, and in the final scene Buzz and Woody are both on the boy's bed, cozily hanging out. Buzz, as the youngest and best of the toys, must endure special hardships. But in the end, he is rewarded with acceptance by his "sibling" toys, including the one who endangered him in the first place. He is even freed from the burden of his space mask, which he can take on and off without harm. Buzz has also been freed from his own difference. It was not only jealousy that separated him from this toy family. His misconception that he was an actual space hero on an alien planet also separated him. By the end, he realizes he is only a toy after all. While that comes as something of a disappointment, it also draws him closer to his fellow toys. They are all in the same boat. He doesn't have to be special anymore in a way that isolates him. The joyful consummation includes not only safety and family harmony but survival of a shared threat—a Christmas scene where the toys (including Buzz) quake in fear that they will be replaced by even glossier toys, a terrible fate that does not come to pass.

While there are similarities between *Toy Story's* plot and Willy's life with his family and his disfiguring injury, these narrative resemblances are not so much discovered as produced through daily family practices that also involve imaginative interpretation, through "making similar to." The first donning of the masks began his identifications with other masked superheroes. But Buzz gets a happy ending that goes beyond that of other superheroes—he finds out that he is just ordinary. He can discard his "mask" and take his place in a toy family, as one among others. The ending that Buzz experiences is one that children with chronic conditions long for—the chance to be just like others. He even gets to be the same as everyone else in a family that—by the end of the film—is characterized by harmony; earlier conflicts among the toys that began when Buzz entered the scene have been happily resolved.

As in *Toy Story*, in which a toy family is united, Willy's family has experienced a happy ending in the sense that—from the perspective of the three parenting women—they have collectively healed themselves from the social wounds caused by Willy's injury. Family ties have strengthened further because of the collective project of taking care of Willy and sharing in the trials and sufferings that his accident has entailed. When the traumatic incident happened, the family was, as his mother puts it, "crippled," but she says that through caring for him they have been "healed." In this regard, the family story's "happy ending" bears a narrative resemblance to the one in *Toy Story*. This resemblance casts a hopeful shadow onto another possible happy ending that is far more tenuous. This is one in which Willy, like Buzz, is no longer "special" but can be a child in the world just like everyone else and in which the family remains united.

I turn to one other example to illustrate the way plots and characters are indigenized to provide a subjunctive language of hope.

THE LITTLE MERMAID AND THE GIRL WITH SPINA BIFIDA

Mima is an eight-year-old girl with severe spina bifida who loves Disney's *The Little Mermaid*. In Mima's case, it was her mother, Zee, who introduced her to *The Little Mermaid* on her first birthday by "reading to her and buying all the characters," as Zee recalls. Mima's entire bedroom is covered with brightly colored pink Little Mermaid stickers. All the main characters adorn the walls. She also has Little Mermaid curtains and Little Mermaid sheets, comforter, and pillowcases—*The Little Mermaid* in surround sound. All this decorating was done not only by Zee but also by her home nurse, who was particularly helpful in putting up the stickers. Just as the Mer princess lives under the sea, encircled by her sea creature friends, so this little girl, who cannot walk and spends much of her day in her bed, lives in a room with sea creatures and mermaids on every side. Like the therapists, nurses, and doctors who remember Willy's identification with Buzz Lightyear, the home health nurse who enthusiastically spends time helping to decorate

Mima's bedroom *Little Mermaid* style affirms Mima's identification with the princess and solidifies her connection not only to the child but also to the mother.

Here too, as with Willy and *Toy Story,* the story of *The Little Mermaid* and Mima's life events—especially those future events her mother most intensely wishes for—have some remarkable parallels. Disney's *Little Mermaid* is a princess whose father rules the Mer people and the seas generally. He commands that the Mer have no traffic with the humans who sail the ocean, and, among their other dangerous attributes, catch and eat fish. His favorite daughter, a rather rebellious sort, secretly covets all things human. She is a sort of anthropologist mermaid, scavenging human artifacts from shipwrecked vessels, relying upon a poorly informed seagull translator to teach her their names and uses. Her "museum" is a vast undersea vault that she hides from her father's sight.

She falls in love with a handsome young sailor, incurring the wrath of her father, who commands Sebastian, a crab with a strong Caribbean accent (and Mima's mother's favorite character), to keep an eye on her. The Mer princess herself has a beautiful voice, as one would expect from a mermaid. In exchange for her voice, she seeks the help of a wicked sea witch with dark powers who promises to give her legs for just three days so she can get the handsome young sailor to marry her. If she cannot persuade her young man to propose to her in that time (during which she will not be able to speak), not only will she lose her legs, but she will never regain her voice. No cure without risk. This is a familiar message for the parents of seriously ill children. Like any good doctor, the sea witch gives her time to think the decision over. The Mer maiden goes home to weigh her options.

This pivotal episode in the movie is mirrored by two events in Mima's and her mother's life. The most obvious parallel between Mima and the mermaid is that neither has legs. The upper half of Mima's body, like that of the Mer princess, is quite strong and developed. Also like the mermaid, Mima has sparkling eyes, a head of pretty dark hair, and an engaging smile. But the lower half of her body seems to barely exist. It is unlikely that she will ever walk. Mima has also lost her voice. This happened several years ago. She has terrible asthma, and when she was younger she had several attacks that were life threatening where she had to be rushed to the hospital. On one occasion when she quit breathing, an emergency tracheotomy was performed to save her life. In *The Little Mermaid,* the tough-minded sea witch "healer" strikes a hard bargain. Uncannily, so did Mima's emergency room doctors who in an even more serious trade took away her voice in exchange for her life.

As for her legs, her mother faced another serious decision regarding surgery that might help Mima's back and her walking. Mima has a wheelchair that she is adept at maneuvering (she can do "wheelies"). She can also crawl. The primary doctor treating Mima has been considering a high-risk surgery to fuse her back, something that Zee hopes might allow her to walk. But such an involved surgery is also life threatening. The arts of the contemporary hospital are not so unlike the dark arts of the sea witch—the possibility of physical transformation but at great potential cost. The physician has given ambivalent messages to Zee about whether this surgery is a realistic possibility and how much it could do to help Mima to walk. Zee recounted a visit with him where they discussed the surgery at length. The physician told her, "I might lose her . . . it's like a fifty-fifty chance. Said it's too risky for her." Zee is considering getting a second opinion because she is not sure if this prognosis says more about the competence or even the moral character of the surgeon than about her daughter's clinical condition. She wonders if the doctor is either "too cowardly" or "too old" to perform such a delicate operation.

For the Little Mermaid it is a different matter. She does make the perilous choice. Things go badly until her father, hearing of his daughter's terrible wager, offers himself up as a sacrifice instead. Finally, after various heroic and daring exploits, the sea witch is out-maneuvered and the handsome young sailor proposes just in time. The movie closes on a wedding scene in which the humans (including the Mer princess, who is presented as a kind of human/Mer hybrid) are married out at sea on a boat with humans on board and the Mer guests holding their (human) heads above water as they watch from the ocean.

The happy ending of *The Little Mermaid* suggests the very plot that Zee desires for her daughter in three important respects. After many trials and close calls, the young mermaid emerges as a young woman who can walk, speak, marry, and bear children (fathered by a handsome husband). This ending speaks to Zee's wishes for her own daughter's future, which she puts succinctly. (She is not the elaborating sort.) She states that she wants her daughter to "walk, to talk," and to be able to "have children." It should be remembered that the entire plot of *The Little Mermaid* turns on the mermaid's acquiring legs, which she does at great risk and only at the price of losing her beautiful voice, a loss that may become permanent. And it is only when her voice returns that she is able to capture the heart of the handsome sailor, who fell in love with her singing long before he met her. Legs, voice, love, children—these are interconnected gifts. The final wedding scene foreshadows by narrative implication that children will follow (this is an old-fashioned story, after all). This promise comes to fruition in *Little Mermaid II*, where the main character is the mermaid's daughter.

The Little Mermaid, however vapid when viewed as yet another hackneyed Disney product, emerges as an immensely versatile forum, a "theater for action" (Appadurai 1996) at the local level. It invites polysemic readings that connect its characters and plot structure in several potent directions simultaneously, and it is this multidimensionality that makes the story so usable for this particular family. The initial movie and its sequel have become part of family life, watched again and again by Zee and her two daughters. *Little Mermaid* scenes show up everywhere in their lives, not only through the myriad artifacts that place Mima in Mer scenes but through key family events (memorialized in numerous family photographs) that have been orchestrated with *The Little Mermaid* in mind. For Mima's first birthday party, her mother invited 150 neighbors, family, and friends to her backyard, which she transformed with an "Under the Sea" theme. This birthday provided an occasion for creating a significant experience, a story in time, and one that will be remembered through pictures and stories for all the girl's life.

In addition to parallels that can be drawn between the plight of Mima's body and the body of the Mer princess, other possibilities for connection reveal something about why her mother identifies so strongly with these movies. Zee admits that *The Little Mermaid* films are her own Disney favorites. When Zee and her two daughters watch the movies together, they develop a shared experience, a shared identification. When asked if her youngest daughter likes "the same parts [of the movie] that you do," she nods her assent, replying, "Her and her sister, yes." Mother and daughters are presented as one. This merger is reinforced by *The Little Mermaid* sequel, a mother-daughter adventure that Zee prefers, in which the Mer princess now has a daughter of her own.

Still other parallels make Disney's *Little Mermaid* films particularly appealing to the family as a whole. Mima's mother is a Belizean immigrant and proud of her Caribbean identity. She and other family members do a great deal of work to maintain it. *The Little Mermaid* handily provides a (playful) emblem of a family, especially in the persona of Sebastian, the Crab, who not only sports a British Caribbean accent but directs an undersea calypso band. These movie scenes suggest lush tropical landscapes that were once, in nostalgic memory, the province of this family. Watching this movie and enacting its scenes in, for example, a child's birthday party with 150 people in attendance serve to produce their unique difference in oblique but powerful ways—members of an English Caribbean diaspora rather than "ordinary" African Americans. Thus once again Disney's Mer princess is indigenized in this family. She emerges as distinctly Belizean in the way the movie is imported into family life. The remaking of the Mer princess into a Caribbean girl is not announced through words or stories told but through the emplotment of a birthday party. The enacted family narrative, a birthday invitation that is also a trip to a tropical, watery paradise, publicly proclaims a family's "true" home, a home invoked in the sea world created in a backyard on an otherwise ordinary low-income Los Angeles street.

Recalling three pivotal elements of narrative (act, agents, and circumstances) introduced earlier in the chapter, how are these reworked in the family "reading" of *The Little Mermaid* in ways that sharpen the narrative symmetry between Mima's life and that of the Mer princess? The most striking example involves the transformation of *The Little Mermaid* into a distinctly Caribbean tale.[6] Disney's Mer princess is "made similar to" Mima in ethnic identification, an ethnicity that, in the eyes of this family, raises her social status as compared to that of (mere) American blacks. This making similar is achieved primarily through Sebastian the Crab—the one character in the movie who is marked as British Caribbean. In the family's reception of the movie, he emerges as a much more significant character than he might otherwise be. Thus his centrality is not an obvious aspect of the film as text but is constructed through family practices of movie consumption. The scenes where he is featured are the ones watched again and again, and the calypso tunes are the ones that the family sings along with. How does this identity shift in character (a Belizean mermaid) shape the meaning of actions and circumstances? It paves the way for seeing these two girls as similar not only in terms of "disability" but in terms of a rather specialized ethnic identity. This connection promotes the suggestion—even if only in imagination—that some version of the Mer princess's fate may one day be shared by Mima.

HOPE AND THE SOCIAL PRACTICE OF FANTASY

The practice of hope, especially the sort of hope that can traverse parent, child, and clinic worlds, may draw upon cultural resources that seem far afield from the business and discourse of clinical care. Global commodities targeted to children can provide a symbolically rich common ground for adults and children. Through localizing strategies, orchestrated by adults as much as children, Disney and other media tales become part of family life, a means for producing family culture. Disability, gender, race, and other significant social markers can be expressed through these commodities. Popular children's films, as reinvented in family life, offer a shared stock of stories known not only to children and parents but to other children (almost) everywhere, and even to other relevant adults, like clinicians, who play a significant role in these children's lives. Because they are so broadly shared, they can be drawn upon, improvised in everyday life. These stories are certainly not scripts, for they are too complex and too fantastical to serve in any literal way as general guides to action. By trafficking in fantasy, they spark the imagination as a resource for envisioning possible lives, possible futures. They are precisely the sort of material necessary for trafficking in the subjunctive (J. Bruner 1986, 1990), and they serve as a "staging ground for action" rather than merely an "escape" (Appadurai 1996:7).

In this chapter I have tried to make a set of arguments. One is that even media products that might appear to reveal globalization at its most worrisome—like Disney's massively popular and influential exports—are taken up in ingenious ways by subaltern groups and remade for local purposes, including the resistance of stigmatized identities. I have focused especially on *reception* as itself a productive act, one that calls upon and provides a resource for imagination. Again, Appadurai's words underscore my point: "More persons throughout the world see their lives through the prisms of the possible lives offered by mass media in all their forms. That is, fantasy is now a social practice; it enters, in a host of ways, into the fabrication of social lives for many people in many societies" (1996:54).

A second argument is that the narrative quality of children's popular films provides audiences possibilities for "making similar to" their own lives through transformations of a story's characters, plot structures, and circumstances. Geographically speaking, the children and families I have come to know as part of this research, many from Los Angeles, abut the Hollywood "dream machine." But they are very far in cultural space. Their practices of appropriation and imagination reveal the flexibility of global narratives to be "rewritten" by those at far social and economic distances from the world and intentions of their producers. Or, as de Certeau might say, their imaginative work reveals how they too produce.

CHAPTER 7

Fleeting Hope

Healing dramas may be powerful, but they may also be ephemeral, momentary bursts of life that cannot be sustained under a harsh clinical gaze. They are fragile moments that are often created, only to be interrupted, ignored, or undermined. The significance of the experiences created is easily lost not only because all lived experience necessarily has a fleeting quality but also because the cultural worlds in which these healing experiences occur do not authorize these kinds of dramas. They have no official status within clinic culture and are not acknowledged as integral to healing.

In chapter 5, I remarked upon Sacks's discovery of how central the image of the journey was to dramatic moments in his own recovery from an injured leg. In depicting his recovery, he tells a story that insists on the centrality of drama to healing, where drama is understood in deeply phenomenological terms, as a transformative experience of the body, one where the body is vividly marked as the "seat" not only of experience but also of self-identity. In the dramatic moments that he describes, his body is transformed from an impediment and obstacle to a site of possibility.

I turn to a puzzle Sacks raises in trying to understand the perspective of his healers. While he finds that his recovery is full of adventures and dramas, his clinicians see things as routine. How can this be? he wonders indignantly. How can they speak of his recovery as "uneventful" when "recovery *is* events, a series of wonderful, unpredictable events . . .

advents, which are births and re-births" (1984:154)? His doctors, nurses, and therapists are unaware of (or find insignificant) what has happened to him. Sacks has his theatrical moments, his astonishing experiences, but he apparently has them all by himself. He experiences dramas—stories in the making—where the professionals see only a mundane, predictable path. When he steals a look at his chart and finds written "uneventful recovery," he concludes that his healers are "mad."

Here I try to explore this "madness" and unpack another kind of paradox central to hope in clinical contexts: its transitory nature. This is especially puzzling when clinicians play such an active role in cultivating it. Whereas Sacks discovers a crucial healing moment on his own, in the examples I have drawn upon, as when Gregory becomes Captain Hook, or Belinda gleefully plays her "Yes I Can" game, clinicians themselves actively assist in the creation of such moments. Sometimes, in other words, clinicians *do* seem to recognize that recovery is constituted through "events" and "rebirths," and this recognition translates into actions that support and foster such recovery dramas. But support is often short-lived, undermined, or aborted altogether. Even when such fostering occurs, the treating practitioner who in one moment helps to create a powerful healing drama may in the next moment deny that she has done so, undo what she has done, or doubt her own wisdom in pursuing such a path.

Herein lies the mystery: Why are clinicians so often ready to relinquish their own good work, even undermining those very healing moments they supported or initiated with patients and families? This chapter investigates the rise and especially the fall of transformative healing dramas. What is it about the nature of clinic practices and discourses that makes this genre so frail, so easily relinquished or neglected? How is it that dominant clinical genres, their institutional embodiment, and the clinical reasoning processes that accompany them work to subvert transformative healing moments?

I take a closer look at the practical reasoning that guides clinical care as a way to explain the "madness" that Sacks speaks of, especially the mysterious inability of clinicians to sustain, to defend, or sometimes even to recognize their own efficacy. In addressing this puzzle, I explore the role of the prevalent mode of reasoning espoused by the canonical genres: a clinical reasoning that obscures those judgments that do not invoke an applied science model of care directed to the diagnosis and treatment of disease. But I also turn to modes of reasoning masked by this espoused model and exposed by poststructuralist practice theorists and their followers. These include the immense importance of "symbolic capital" in shaping quality of care, biotechnology's place in generating greater symbolic capital for certain clinical professions vis-à-vis others and in reproducing a particular hierarchy of clinical care, and the influence of expert-driven "pastoral reasoning" in directing the decision making of clinicians.

As a first illustration, I return to Andrena's relationship with her child's oncologist, Dr. Branden, to illustrate the tragic manner in which she perceived him to "abandon" her as her daughter grew increasingly ill and medical treatments were withdrawn.

DR. BRANDEN DISAPPEARS

After eighteen months of intensive treatment, Belinda's chemotherapy was discontinued. She no longer saw Dr. Branden or made her biweekly trips to the hospital. I turn to the last moments of Belinda's life to explore the way clinicians abandoned a healing drama. In particular, the "disappearance" of the oncologist underscores the limitations of canonical healing genres. Unlike the genre of transformative journey, which can promote a changing picture of hope and a changing anticipatory narrative, the canonical genres lack this imaginative flexibility. When it becomes clear that no biomedical happy ending can be realized, hope is lost altogether. By the spring of 1999, despite all the efforts of Dr. Branden and the medical team, Belinda's cancer began to spread. For Dr. Branden, there was nothing else he could do "medically." For Andrena, caring for her critically ill daughter very centrally involved embarking on her own moral quest, one where she might have to be strong enough even to bear the "bad news" that her child was indeed dying.

Andrena expected that health professionals—especially Dr. Branden, who trafficked in death every day—would make the same journey she did, shifting from a view of healing as curing to one in which they accepted that despite everything they had tried, it was "God's call." She did not expect Belinda's clinicians to share her religious beliefs. But she had come to think that she and Dr. Branden were "partnering up" in this terrible voyage and that as a partner he would be there for the entire trip, even, as she put it, "through the death part."

Being there might have taken several forms. At best, Dr. Branden might have come to the funeral. But Andrena was not asking for this.

At the least, he could have been the one to bring her the terrible news, namely, that there was nothing more he or the hospital could do to keep Belinda alive. Instead, he delegated this task to the case nurse. In an interview about a year after Belinda's death, Andrena talked frankly about how hard it had been when he suddenly disappeared, exiting at the most difficult time of all. Here she reports in vivid detail the fateful conversation she had with the nurse case manager about her child's impending death.

> *Cheryl:* Was it Dr. Branden who finally told you that the tumor had spread?
>
> *Andrena:* No, it was Sarah, the case manager. It was right before Christmas, and they didn't know if we wanted to stay there or go home and do hospice. Because she [the nurse case manager], at that time she said, "Well, there's nothing they could do now. Um, she's not gonna make it." I asked her, "Well, how long?" She said, "Maybe three, six months." You know. And she lasted exactly three.

Andrena explains why this conversation with the nurse, one she thought she should have had with Dr. Branden, felt like such a betrayal. She moves beyond her own experience, speaking as part of a collective for other parents who have had this same experience—doctors who "disappear" at the end.

> *Andrena:* That's what they [the doctors] do. That's bad. Because that's when the parent really wants to talk to the doctor. Because the doctor's been following their child, and they feel that only the doctor could be the one to tell them what's going on. They don't wanna see someone else come to bring bad news. They want their doctor to be there so they can even *(she pauses)* maybe cry to their doctor. And tell their doctor how they feel, you know? I mean, I enjoyed Sarah while I was there with her, you know, as the case manager, but I wanted Dr. Branden to tell me. I didn't want somebody else. 'Cause I felt like he was running. I felt like he didn't wanna come to me and tell me, which I felt he was the only one that I would believe. I felt he should've been the one.
>
> *Cheryl:* Sure.
>
> *Andrena:* I said, "Where is he?" That's the first thing I asked. She [the nurse manager] said, "He's on vacation." And I didn't want nobody else to tell me nothing.
>
> *Cheryl:* Yeah.
>
> *Andrena:* So I think the doctors run away, or say that they're away. And when someone else told me that that happened to them, I said, "Oh, so it's just a routine."

Andrena tried in other ways to have some final conversation with Dr. Branden. She wrote to him and telephoned as well. But she never heard back.

> *Andrena:* I sent Dr. Branden a card, you know . . . I just sent him a card, you know, thanking him for being, doing what he could do for Belinda and everything. I left him a message, but I didn't hear from him any more.

She tries to puzzle out why he would not have contacted her. She is stunned by what she perceives as a "heartless" end to their partnership. She wonders if there is some institutional policy that dictates against it, a kind of institutional coldheartedness. The message she receives from this is that they are saying, "Forget you!"

> *Andrena:* I don't know, maybe they're not supposed to speak with any of the parents. But, you know, it sure would make the parents feel better. And I've heard that from a couple of other parents, you know, they just feel like when your daughter, you know, your son, whoever, is gone, it's like they say, forget you! And the part, the worst part is, it makes the parents feel so bad when you know, um, when you feel like nobody cares, you know? It's heartless.
>
> *Cheryl:* Yeah.
>
> *Andrena:* It's a coldhearted feeling when the parents, you know, after they spend so much time there, you know, you would think that they would have some kind of feelings.

She continues to mull over this unexpected and abrupt withdrawal by the doctor. She offers another hypothesis. Perhaps it isn't a cold-hearted hospital policy but an understandable vulnerability in the doctors themselves.

> *Andrena:* Maybe, you know, it could be that they need therapy, too. . . . It's like um, guys in the war, you know. After seein' so many dead people, they need therapy because they have flashbacks. I don't know. Maybe the doctors could need therapy, too.

Dr. Branden's disappearance disturbs Andrena partly because of its failure to fit the healing narrative she believed she was sharing with him, that they were living out together. This was one created from clinical visits I described earlier where he and Belinda played the "Yes I Can" game. From her perspective, such a visit was a powerful short story in which the doctor was both a medical professional, a practicing scientist, and a healer of a different sort, one who could join with her in delighting in Belinda's love of play, her joy in defiance, her affectionate nature. This was a doctor, the only kind one she could trust, who saw Belinda as a little girl, not just a "cancer kid." Their trading of family stories and his ability to participate in a family game revealed a level of attachment that Andrena associated with good care. She was not simply gauging a "compassion" factor. This was an important indicator of what kind of medical care her daughter was receiving, whether treatments were being withheld because she was on public aid or because her daughter was African American and therefore less valuable. Did she lack the symbolic capital to ensure the best care?

Dr. Branden's failure to see things through to the end or even to deliver the bad news completely disrupts the healing narrative Andrena thought she was living. His actions violate the ending she anticipated, even what she thought would be the worst possible ending, the one where her child would die. In this narrative violation, a new and terrible fear emerges. Has she misjudged him all along? If he deserts her at this point, and does not even contact her long after the funeral when she tries to reach him, did he ever really care for her daughter? And if he did not, did Andrena do all she could to get her child good care? Can she still hold to the healing story she told at the funeral, the one where her daughter had everything she needed in her short life? Andrena is forced into a retrospective mistrust that she can never quite relinquish.

For his part, Dr. Branden believed he had come to the (unhappy) end of the healing drama with Belinda because he had come to the end of what he could do *technically*: the "battle" with cancer was lost. He had fought as long and hard as he could, but ultimately he was vanquished. His work as an oncologist was done. While Andrena might very well be right that he "ran away" because he could not emotionally bear the pain of Belinda's death, he was also acting in a manner congruent with clinic culture, in which healing was identified with what medical technology could bring to bear. What was the "diagnosis" he would be treating at the moment the battle with disease was over?

As I noted in earlier chapters, within the canonical dramas of biomedicine clinicians emerge as rational instrumentalists who strategically work to deploy a means-ends rationality directed to repair bodies, attack disease, and solve mysteries. This reasoning process is justified by an empiricist and essentialist understanding of reality and the belief that the ultimate reality one is dealing with is biological.[1] The body emerges as a thing apart from its human significance. In Western society generally, the rational and instrumental, in which medicine is squarely placed, are separated from the symbolic and affective. As a rational and instrumental practice, medicine appears to discover natural truths that transcend the particularities of context (Comaroff 1982:49).

This dissociation occurs in an everyday way as medical professionals find ways to routinize their practice and thus, metaphorically at least, bring the unruly and frightening world of illness under control. By nature, illness is unpredictable, and much of medicine is fraught with uncertainty (Hunter 1991). Medicine's goal to control illness, or at least give the appearance of control, is well recognized,[2] and the elaboration of medical technology and its attendant rituals are prime means to do so.[3] Biomedicine's tremendous focus on technology as the source of solutions to disease reinforces a practice in which much more attention is given to means than ends (Gordon 1988).

A commitment to scientific neutrality creates a very deep and baneful divide that persists within clinical care—the division between the ethical and the technical. This separation underlies the ambivalence clinicians display toward any view that links healing to personal and interpersonal transformation. While caring or well-intentioned clinicians would, of course, not deny that it is people who suffer and people they treat, the canonical genres into which they are socialized train them to sideline or trivialize this "human" aspect of care. It may be important, but it is ultimately not an essential element of their particular expert knowledge. In Byron Good and Mary-Jo DelVecchio Good's (1993) study of medical school students, we can see precisely how this perception is cultivated. Medical school involves socialization into "becoming doctors," propelled by powerful and dramatic experiences (like anatomy lab) that precipitate a new understanding of the body, one that disconnects body from person. This disconnection is critical to the *drama* of the canonical genres and can mask the powerful work clinicians do that falls outside these dramas. Clinicians are often surprisingly oblivious to how consequential their actions can be, dismissing beautifully orchestrated partnerships they have created by describing them as just a matter of being "kind" to distraught parents or frightened children or simply not noticing when they are effective. Sometimes, as in the following example, they have no authoritative language to challenge the decisions made by higher-status clinicians.[4]

FELICIA AND THE RAVEN-HAIRED POCAHONTAS

One winter day I (along with my research colleague, Mary Lawlor) observed a session in which an occupational therapist, Penny, was treating a girl about thirteen or fourteen years old. We will call her Felicia. Special educators at Felicia's school had referred her for treatment at this outpatient clinic. Once a week Felicia was bussed from school to the hospital for therapy. The therapist told us in a later interview something of the diagnostic history that had brought Felicia to occupational therapy. This included leukemia when she was eight or nine (now in remission), seizure disorders, and a fuzzy psychiatric diagnosis, which was variously labeled by clinicians and teachers as an "oppositional defiant disorder" or "conduct disorder." Penny was to specifically address the child's delays in fine motor and visual motor skills. Felicia's teachers especially wanted the therapist to work on her handwriting, which was very messy.

At the time of the session, the therapist had known Felicia for about two years. They had a very close relationship. Felicia was the only one in her school who got to go to occupational therapy, and this made her feel special. She also enjoyed what they did in occupational therapy, which was mostly a lot of craft projects and some handwriting and computer writing work. While Felicia missed a lot of school, she never missed Fridays. The therapist said that she would "always beg her father on Thursday night to make sure that he woke her up for Friday because she didn't want to miss O.T."

Here is the scene we observed when we first met Felicia. In she walks to the occupational therapy treatment room, a bouncy and rather large girl, a little unkempt but with a tremendously friendly smile. Penny and Felicia initially struggle over which activity to do in therapy. Penny offers Felicia the option of one among several possible prepackaged sand painting kits. The outside boxes show pictures of the finished paintings (all Disney characters from various movies), and Felicia pores carefully over each one. This initial scene between Penny and Felicia is keyed playfully but with a serious undertone, in which the therapist is trying to speed Felicia along, clearly with an eye to their limited time. Felicia makes a great show of indecisiveness and even seems to be teasing Penny. "Jeez, don't rush me!" she says with a great laugh and a conspiratorial grin to the two unknown observers huddled in the corner watching the scene with their notebooks open. Finally things settle down, and we see that, at the therapist's urging, they are going to do a sand painting of Pocahontas. This Pocahontas, in the finished illustration featured on the cover, is a very pretty slim girl of about sixteen with many brightly colored birds circling her head like a kind of halo. All about her is a very blue sky. Penny and Felicia settle at a small table with their kit and prepare to get started. They immediately contest just how they are going to organize the task. Shall they line up the colored packets of sand by their numbers (Penny's preference), or by those that just seem to fit together (Felicia's scheme)?

Ten or fifteen minutes into the session, things get going. Felicia gradually becomes absorbed, pouring the sand with painstaking care and surveying her work with a critical eye. She appears to have forgotten her audience entirely. She is silent, intent, crafting her picture, with occasional guidance from the therapist. A few minutes later, they color Pocahontas's hair, which makes up a large patch of the picture. This is glossy, shiny black hair, silky and long. The therapist says to Felicia, "She's very pretty." They both agree. Penny then tells her, "She has hair like yours!" The therapist is right. Felicia may not be the beautiful Disneyfied Pocahontas, but she has her hair exactly—the same silky blue-black hair of this fairytale girl surrounded by these lovely birds.

I could suddenly see that this session was a place where pictures were made. These were not most importantly literal ones but rather imaginative ones where images were created and negotiated. The activities of Penny and Felicia created a sort of image, a kinesthetic image of concentration and focus required to craft something Felicia found worth creating. Felicia shifted from being a bouncy but tendentious girl to one who concentrated with her head bent, completely focused on her task—a girl who had the skills and desire to create something that brought her pleasure, someone who could sit still long enough to do a good job.

And the picture itself, however foolish and fantastical, offered another image. It was not just any picture but a picture of a girl not so much older than Felicia, and with that same abundance of rich black hair. When she smiled, Felicia even gave off something of Pocahontas's cheery brilliance. (In fact, there was something preferable about the impishness of Felicia's grin when compared to the blank beauty of the Walt Disney character.) But look at Pocahontas! Loved by all, even the birds. Free to wander under a clear sky.

Penny worried a little that she allowed Felicia to select therapeutic activities that were "seven-, eight-, nine-year-old-type things . . . if you compare her to other girls fourteen and fifteen, you know, they'd be more into music or whatever." Yet she helped Felicia to create magical and pretty worlds, magical girls like Pocahontas, in these moments of therapy time, which had come to mean so much to Felicia. Though Penny didn't quite seem to realize it, what got created here was not so much a picture as an *event,* an event that signaled possibility. Here was a little drama with qualities associated with healing rituals: a multimedia, symbolically freighted, dramatic, and compelling social creation. The resonance between this present moment and Felicia's past and future emerged even more clearly after interviews with the therapist.

This session was a short story in a larger life story still very much unfolding, whose ending was not at all certain. Compare Pocahontas's story to the fate Penny feared for Felicia. Penny stated that Felicia had "self-esteem problems." Felicia spoke of herself as looking "yucky." Penny told a terrifying story of a meeting between school professionals, hospital therapists, and parents when she met Felicia's mother for the first time. She described her as a tall stern woman who "yelled" at all the school and therapy professionals, told them they didn't understand her daughter, and announced that she was keeping Felicia for home schooling rather than sending her to school. Felicia sat in a corner and hung her head during this meeting. When Penny had to leave early, Felicia begged to go with her. So Penny took her out of the meeting.

The therapist also recounted her final session with Felicia (the week after the one we observed), when they just went to sit and talk. Felicia, for the first time, talked about her home life in real detail. She, her mother and father, her two-year-old niece, and her two brothers all live in a one-bedroom apartment. The therapist, hand held over her heart, offered her picture of Felicia in a few years. Felicia was already the primary caretaker for her niece, a two-year-old left by Felicia's older sister, who was never home. The therapist imagined her as the designated family babysitter, eating potato chips and sitting in front of the TV, year in and year out. This was her dark, fearful vision.

Penny was simultaneously helping Felicia address a series of discrete difficulties she faced (for example, paying attention, doing a job well, remembering things, and coordinating her physical movements) and helping her with a larger project. Penny labeled it "building her self-esteem," and certainly that was part of it. But perhaps we could also say that Penny believed Felicia might lack a hopeful picture of her future self, one that would help guide her in finding the best possible life for herself. Put differently, we might say that Felicia lacked a picture of herself that would help her to see her own possibilities and strengths. Pocahontas might not be a very realistic alternative, but the ability to create Pocahontas, to make with your hands a beautiful magical mirror, such an experience may beget other sorts of creations. One need not accept Penny's version of Felicia's life, but there are many indicators, just in the single session offered here, that this was "an experience" for Felicia. It was not a singular momentous event, like the one described by Sacks, but in its quiet way it presented a striking image that Felicia just might take home.

On the one hand, Penny was confident that she offered something important and unique to Felicia. She told us that for Felicia she had become "that one special person to do something with." Penny, who was in her early twenties at the time and had a girlish air, believed Felicia saw her as a kind of "friendly older sister." Felicia had also treated her as a protector on occasion—during the one time Penny met Felicia's mother at a team meeting, a woman whose anger frankly frightened Penny, Felicia shrank away, grabbing Penny's hand for comfort.

CLINICAL HIERARCHIES AND THE FRAGILITY OF HEALING

Where is the precariousness in this healing drama? Penny lacked conviction that her work had anything to do with healing. She agreed with team members that Felicia should be discharged from therapy. In the end, Penny did not know how to defend her work with Felicia. Perhaps it really was, as she put it, "just a social thing." After all, she readily admitted, Felicia's handwriting had never improved in two years, and that was a main treatment goal of their work. She spoke sadly of the plans she and Felicia had made about future therapy together.

> We also did a lot of work on the computer because her handwriting was so sloppy and there really wasn't, that was not going to change. That had been worked on for three years and in school every day. So we started working on the computer and doing typing and hoping that maybe this could be a way that in the future she could be working and, you know, doing a vocational program or something. So we had talked about doing, making a newspaper which I had started with another one of the day school kids that she knew about.

Not only was Felicia discharged from therapy, but Felicia's mother decided to take her out of the school program. She told the professional team she wanted to give Felicia home schooling instead, a decision that deeply disturbed Penny. In our final interview with Penny, tears came to her eyes as she spoke of Felicia's future. She was clearly haunted by this case. A year later, Penny decided to leave pediatric practice because she found it just too emotionally difficult.

Penny might have strongly advocated that Felicia stay in therapy, particularly since she was going to be home schooled and would lose most other contact with the world outside her family. Perhaps Penny might not have won this battle, but she didn't even try. Furthermore, despite her terrible visions for Felicia's future, she seemed to find her colleagues' recommendations for Felicia's discharge reasonable. Why? We could go a certain way in answering this by pointing toward biomedicine's canonical genres, which define illness in narrow diagnostic terms and identify rehabilitation with well-specified procedures that can be judged against clearly observable, ideally measurable gains in function. But these genres are also embedded within institutional practices and hierarchies of expertise that consolidate truth and power, exercising surveillance upon the lesser experts by those with higher-status authority. Thus this example also speaks to the hierarchy of diagnostic categories, even in this comparatively low-status contest: even "improved handwriting" trumps "improved self-esteem." Clinical creators of healing dramas very often abandon them because of the organizing role of the diagnosis in framing what constitutes appropriate treatment. In the clinical world, some diagnoses are more "real" and more deserving of clinical attention than others. The power of any particular diagnosis is not necessarily linked to its impact on a patient's overall health but rather based on its symbolic (and economic) capital.

Another kind of hierarchy is also critical here: the power and ranking of the diagnostician who has "awarded" the diagnosis to a particular patient. Technology and specialized training play a key part in determining the symbolic capital of any given diagnosis. In their dystopic portraits of clinical practice, many anthropologists have repeatedly underscored the technocratic nature of Western biomedicine and the insidious ill effects of health care built around such technology (Browner and Press 1995). One structural consequence of this technology-centric vision of healing is that psychologists and therapists who administer comparatively "low-tech" medicine assume much lower status than, for example, surgeons who treat some of the highest-status and most technologically intricate clinical diseases. Furthermore, a reductive emphasis on the canonical genres means that treatment goals in rehabilitation tend to emphasize "fixing" or improving body parts rather then the subtle task of instigating personal or social transformation.

What, following Foucault, one might call "pastoral reasoning" enters in a subtle fashion as higher-status clinicians function as both clinical and governmental gatekeepers in determining who gets care and who doesn't. Canonical biomedical genres carry moral imperatives. It is not simply that one has the technical capacity to repair a broken body/ machine or attack a virulent cancer. One has the moral imperative to do so. Clinicians are routinely called upon to make decisions about which patients "deserve care" and which do not. They find themselves assigned the task of the gatekeeper, deciding who will receive services and who will not partly on the basis of interpretations and judgments about the moral worth of patients' lives.[5] The pastoral reasoning evident in this case has also been demonstrated elsewhere in this book, as in the clinical staff's dilemmas and discussions concerning what do to about Ron and his daughter Ronetta in chapter 5.

Interestingly, many rehabilitation therapists seem to reject canonical versions of biomedical hope when they are informally interviewed "off the record." It is very common that when they describe what they think really matters about their interventions they will stress the importance of using therapy time to encourage dramatic transformations in the perspectives and practices of patients and family members. But even those rehabilitation therapists who are particularly adept at encouraging children to engage in highly creative activities, embedding exercises designed to "redirect eye attention" or "improve gross motor coordination" within imaginative scenarios that delight the children, will often speak dismissively of these efforts in subsequent interviews. "You know, with kids, you really have to motivate them or they won't work in therapy," they explain with some embarrassment when they have resorted to creative and playful treatment programs.[6]

Higher-status practitioners like physicians who themselves find creative ways to connect with children and families sometimes critique subordinates for spending too much time "just playing" with children instead of "getting the work done" of doing the prescribed exercises. Talking and playing are typically set against exercises, procedures, and other "real work" features of clinical practice in such a way that the former are perceived to take time away from the latter. The institutional hierarchy sets rehabilitation therapists (with their concern over comparatively low-status diagnostic problems) against much more powerful professionals. One of the surgeons in our study, for example, world renowned for his skills in performing notoriously intricate brachial plexus injury surgeries, readily admitted that rehabilitation therapies were critical to the functional outcome of such surgeries. This surgeon remarked that he was continually waging a battle with the rehabilitation therapists to put in more of their time doing "stretching" and other exercises directed at the injured site rather than spending their time "merely playing" with children. He was expressing a concern that therapists focus on goals directly tied to the surgeries. In this sense, surgeons are dependent upon the actions of the less high-ranking professionals and patients themselves for their surgeries to be successful. He stated, with some resignation, that good recovery routinely depends "70 percent on rehabilitation" and "30 percent on surgery," no matter how skilled the physician.

So while from a therapist's perspective emotional disabilities may prove the greatest health risk, from a more powerful institutional perspective the success of much more prestigious interventions like surgery or the improvement of measurable school-based skills like handwriting takes precedence. Therapists may see these as interrelated issues. They cannot get to the higher-ranking diagnostic problem without "treating the behavior," they will complain. But if institutionally legitimated issues improve markedly or fail to improve, as in Penny's situation, then diffuse social behavioral diagnoses or vague fears that a life will not be lived well (for example, that the patient will be reduced to the family babysitter) cannot be used to argue for continued treatment.

Thus clinicians like Penny who facilitate powerful healing dramas readily discharge the children rather than make the case to colleagues or families for continued treatment. Short stays and early discharges are, of course, readily traced to a reimbursement system largely out of the hands of individual clinicians. But this economic pact does not fully explain things. It is not simply that patients are discharged too soon; the irony is that clinicians consistently abandon their own powerful efforts. That is, their own representations of their practice are characteristically deeply ambivalent. Furthermore, their clinical actions and decisions are often marked by this same ambivalence.

The link between healing and technology in Western biomedical practices becomes evident in a different sense when one looks at those health care practices where the "hands-on" skill of the professional is the primary tool for treatment. Biomechanical metaphors apply not merely to the body of the patient but to the healer as well. Rehabilitation therapists are often viewed, and sometimes view themselves, as easily interchangeable providers of technical interventions. Key decisions about intervention are often made apart from what the actual healer, like Penny, might determine as necessary, as when a therapist "inherits" a patient who has already been marked as ready for discharge. Canonical dramas are played out by a host of clinical "characters," and the heroic is often reserved for actions of the higher-status clinician. For example, take the orthopedic surgeon I quoted earlier, with his renowned surgical expertise. His surgeries have attracted television coverage, but the rehabilitation that follows has not, since it merely serves as a routine conclusion to these television-worthy dramas.

Perhaps the most powerful impediment to the recognition and cultivation of healing dramas within the modern clinic has to do with the disconnection between what healers like Penny believe, in an almost private way, to be important for a given patient and what they feel they can legitimately claim to know. Their claims to authoritative knowledge do not include the capacity to redirect treatment to tackle diagnostically diffuse emotional and behavioral problems of their patients, especially not when treatment looks, as Penny remarks dejectedly, like "just a social thing." Turf issues and a myriad of other institutional factors stand between these healers and their own "personal knowledge," to use Michael Polanyi's (1974) important term. In such situations, Western biomedicine, with its particular claims to authoritative knowledge, undermines confidence not only in the embodied knowledge of sufferers but also in that of the healers themselves.[7] Yet the cultivation of healing dramas in which, for instance, Felicia can reveal her wit and charm demands that Penny draw upon her own embodied knowledge.

When Sacks's experiences of recovery are not shared by his healers, he improves anyway. He recovers both his leg and his life. As it turns out, his healing is not dependent upon his healers' recognition of the dramas of recovery. Felicia, Belinda, and the other children I speak about in this book are often not so lucky. They are not blessed with the economic resources or the symbolic capital that Sacks has at his disposal, and their injuries and illnesses are far graver. Felicia and Belinda *do* encounter healers who seem to recognize, at some level, that healing in the world of chronic illness and disability requires the creation of significant moments, moments that reveal possible worlds and possible selves worth striving for. But from the clinical side, these dramas are constructed within the confines of institutional worlds. Such worlds largely constrain these professionals' vision of their task. When healing dramas are not sufficiently prized, healing may falter or fail altogether. For children and parents, this abandonment by professionals threatens the possibility of emplotting lives such that these dramatic moments in clinical time become episodes in a larger and longer-lasting drama of healing, one that can even transcend the death of a child.

I might seem to suggest here that if clinicians could only manage to embrace the idea that healing is a transformative journey, the dilemmas, conflicts, and dystopian scenarios that so often arise between clinicians and patients with chronic conditions would be resolved. But this is far from true. It is more accurate to say that adopting any version of this genre would confront clinicians with a practice of hope more promising, more paradoxical, and more tragic than any of the hopes governed by the canonical genres.

CHAPTER 8

Narrative Phenomenology and the Practice of Hope

In this concluding chapter, I briefly summarize some of the overarching arguments that I have worked to make throughout the book. But I also return to two people who have served as central protagonists: Andrena and Ronetta. It seems appropriate to conclude a book in which I have insisted on the importance of the experience-near, the eventful, and the personal with an epilogue that takes us back to people's lives.

HOPE IN THE BORDERLANDS

I have concentrated on hope as connected to one key task: creating borderland communities between clinicians, patients, and families. The cultivation of hope depends upon the politics of this relational work, however temporary, however tenuous. When partnerships break down, as they routinely do, or are never formed at all, it is difficult for either families or clinicians to create and sustain hope for the children under their care. Thus the sociality of creating hope remains a very pressing and immediate concern of families, clinicians, and, especially as they get older, the children themselves. And in an effort to create strong border communities, families (and sometimes the children too) devise any number of inventive ways to cultivate bonds or to seek out new border communities that may serve them better.

I have made a number of claims in this book about what a narrative phenomenology of practice offers to an investigation of how hope is denied, cultivated, and subverted in clinical border zones. I have suggested that a dramatistic lens provides a way to think about practices and practical action that connects hope as a highly personal and local matter to larger frames of action, including national discourses and practices, even the global circulation of goods. It allows us to give an account of historically particular social interactions and even personal experiences, while situating these extremely situated events and experiences within larger political and social frameworks. It connects small-scale dramas—particular historical events as experienced by particular historical actors in particular contexts—to larger social histories. It offers us a way to connect history writ small to history writ large, to draw together grand histories with highly personal ones. It can even say something about the cosmopolitan nature of social life.

To turn it the other way round, narrative phenomenology allows us to think suggestively, and in ethnographic detail, about large-scale historical events as these are lived and experienced by local actors situated somewhere. It allows us to consider the macro and the structural from personal perspectives. This ability to offer a rich portrait from the actors' point of view is one of narrative's most important possibilities. A narrative framework is so well suited to moving between the highly particular and the large-scale in a *practice-oriented way* because narratives show us life in process; social life emerges not as a completed act, or as the mere enactment of a pregiven cultural logic, but as the local improvisation of everyday actors. This processual and performative picture of human life allows us to see how people draw upon cultural resources in actions directed to trying to get things done that they care about, to further their commitments. Or in the narrative language I have drawn upon—they try to make certain kinds of stories come true and thwart other possible stories. Furthermore, and I think this is one of narrative's most important potentials, such a lens can help us to look at social life not just as a past flowing into the present but from the perspective of the future—life as imaginatively constructed, as hoped for, as dreaded, a vulnerable thing. A narrative phenomenology offers an especially powerful vantage point from which to see how the past and present are saturated by dreams—and nightmares—of the future.

In placing a theoretical emphasis upon the drama of interpersonal life, I have examined the way that actors act and interpret what others are up to by placing actions within presumed narrative contexts in which these actions make sense. Through such active emplotment, time itself takes on narrative shape and particular events become meaningful to actors as episodes in unfolding stories. Such sense making is part and parcel of practical action, helping to guide what future actions might be possible or reasonable and assessing what potential future stories could be furthered or thwarted by one's actions. This active emplotment is always culturally informed, I have also contended. Emergent, acted narratives, while improvised to fit context, are by no means invented from scratch. Actors draw upon cultural resources to interpret what sort of stories they are in and to imagine what sort of stories they might be able to create. Actors draw upon, and in turn reinvent, a continually changing stock of available stories and story types. These narrative artifacts do not provide rules for action so much as imaginative possibilities for "reading" the actions of oneself and others.

In introducing a narrative phenomenology of hope, I have attempted the conceptual task of creating a space of hope that neither forecloses the possibility of personal and social transformation nor invokes an optimism that relies on an ideal of cure or the emergence of new "regimes of truth."[1] The practice of hope is certainly very much a structural and political matter as well. It has been essential to illuminate the everyday workings of institutions of power and the insidious ways inequalities and domination are routinely produced there. The institutional features that render hope fleeting in a clinical setting are not peculiar to clinical life, with its particular hierarchies and teams of experts. Governmentality and the policing of experts extend throughout our social worlds. They are part and parcel of everyday experience, of social practice, of subjectivity itself. I have tried to consider social structure, with all of its oppressive force, as necessary to an analysis of hope but to consider it in a way that does not eclipse the struggles of people to create hope in their lives.

In fact, it has been quite striking in this research project how many parents have become political activists—unwillingly or unexpectedly, as they have said—precisely because of their experiences trying to create border partnerships with clinicians. Out of these personal experiences, many have come to recognize that neither they nor their clinicians can improve health care or solve health inequities without also addressing the larger political and economic forces that shape the delivery of health care. More than one parent has talked about her trips to the state legislature in Sacramento to advocate for more funding or social services for children with a particular disease. "It is not just about my child," parents will say. "We have to do something about all the children who are suffering from this disease." I have not undertaken an analysis of this evolution of hope from the merely personal or familial to the explicitly political in this book. (It is the subject of a subsequent book I am currently writing.) However, it is worth mentioning that many families in this study see the connection between the personal, the interpersonal, and the structural. Through their experiences seeking health care for their children, many come to reframe hope in ways that are not only personal but also political and structural.

We cannot get at any deep, practical understanding of the forces and conditions of power or possibility without—at a theorized level and not merely as case studies and illustrations—following them through the lives of people whom we come, as researchers and as readers, to in some sense know. There is a need to think about hope and its paradoxes without reducing it to a product of discursive practices, to recognize it as a force for personal and social change emergent in interpersonal events, in personal and family lives, in communities.

TRANSFORMATIVE JOURNEYS AND LIVES IN SUSPENSE

Throughout this book, I have offered many humble moments (often of clinical sessions) to explore the practice of hope from discursive, personal, and above all event-centered perspectives. The long-term nature of the research my colleagues and I have carried out has also allowed me to consider hope in horizons that stretch across a substantial span of someone's life. It is when we look at people's lives "in motion" (Lawlor 2003, 2004) and over time that the genre of "transformative journey" is most revealing. In fact, it seems impossible to speak of hope in a person-centered way without invoking the image of life as a journey. This image takes on a particular cultural cast for African Americans who come with a history rooted in slavery. Scholars like Du Bois and West have noted the cultural significance of that very first terrible voyage across the Atlantic as formative of how hope and resilience have been fashioned in the African American experience. The "metaphorical association of black hearts, black people, and black culture with water (the sea or a river) runs deep in black artistic expression. . . . Black striving resides primarily in movement and motion, resilience and resistance against the paralysis of madness and the stillness of death" (West, quoted in Gates and West 1996:82–83). In this concluding chapter, I return to two of the people I have spoken about in earlier chapters to consider this journey and to suggest what can be seen about hope as it changes over time. How does the practice of creating community within clinical settings also undergo its own transformations?

First, a word about Andrena, the person who has functioned as such a primary character. One might imagine that upon the death of her child and her sense of abandonment by the pediatric oncologist Andrena would have had nothing more to do with the hospital and the clinicians who had cared for her daughter. But the opposite turned out to be the case. She drew upon her experience as a source of a different kind of hope—an activist hope. Perhaps she could help make things better for other parents whose children were also suffering, or even dying, from cancer. Not only did she join the local volunteer cancer association at her hospital, she created her own "Belinda Foundation," trying to raise money nationally to help out parents whose children were seriously ill. Her idea was that parents themselves were desperate for support in ways clinicians and policy makers might overlook. They needed not only better information about what to expect but also small but crucial services and reminders of the everyday. She brought Mother's Day baskets to the hospital for parents who were staying with their children, for example, and even washed clothes and ran errands for parents who did not want to leave their child's side.

It is not that Andrena moved past her own grief or resolved her misgivings about how well she had managed this "border-crossing" work that she had come to pride herself on when Belinda was still alive. But she tried to use her experience to create a role for herself as culture broker with other parents less familiar with how to navigate in the hospital world. Thus her practice of hope shifted after her daughter died. She began taking a nurse's course through night classes at the local high school and convinced her surviving daughter (Belinda's half sister) to do the same. While Andrena did not ultimately pursue this career, her daughter, in fact, completed training and got a job at the same hospital where Belinda had been treated and Andrena volunteered.

RONETTA'S TRAVEL TALE

I conclude this book with one final travel story. This time I shift perspective, examining the cultivation of hope as a border practice that children, too, undertake. Knowing families for such a long time has meant that increasingly some of the children have emerged as the primary culture brokers between clinical and family life. I introduce

Ronetta at the age of seventeen and eighteen, the child I described in chapter 4. At the time of the session with the physical therapy aide that was the focus of that chapter, she was nearly thirteen years old. At that point she had been in the hospital almost continuously for two years. These lengthy hospitalizations, it may be remembered, were precipitated by a severe stroke that occurred when she was eleven, in which, she tells us many years later, she "almost died."

A few months after that difficult session with the physical therapy aide, we lost track of her and her family. In fact, we did not see them for four years. They had moved and we couldn't get a forwarding address or phone number. For reasons of confidentiality, we were reluctant to approach clinicians who had treated Ronetta to find out what had happened to this family. I assumed the worst, that Ronetta had been taken out of her father's custody and put into foster care. Perhaps Ron was even in jail, I speculated glumly. I knew he had a prison record (though, as was common for many of the families, he had alluded to it in the vaguest terms—having spent time "upstate" or "away" or "out of town"). I had an unshakable image of Ronetta, still trapped in a body that was "shaped like a chair," still in constant pain, feeling abandoned by both her parents.

Then one day in 2007 Ron called and said that he had missed being part of our project. He seemed to have the idea that we had "given up" on him and sounded a bit aggrieved that we had been out of touch for so long. He and his daughter rejoined the study, and to our astonishment things had turned out remarkably differently than anticipated. Ronetta had developed into a strikingly poised and elegant young woman, far different from the girl I remembered from her intensive hospital days. She had learned to walk again and had been able to return to school full time. In the spring of 2008 she graduated from high school. In 2008 and 2009, she began attending a local community college. Her goal was to become a pediatric hematologist so that she could, as she said, take care of kids like her because she knew how miserable it was to be a child living in a hospital.

I turn to a consideration of her experiences of what it had been like to live in a hospital world with a chronic illness, what it had meant to be part of a troubled family, how she had learned to become an adept border crosser in health care worlds, and how race and class had shaped her experience of her illness. Ronetta's own travels as she reached young adulthood say a great deal about what it means to struggle for a life worth living despite the uncertainties and vulnerabilities of living with a chronic illness. Her travels, which had included regular trips to the hospital for transfusions and to manage pain crises, also speak to how her own hope had been powerfully shaped by her skills at creating communities with the clinicians who treated her. The key dramas of her life had had every bit as much to do with these skills and this relationship building as with her biological family relationships. In fact, in her case, the boundary between them had truly blurred. She had created a hybrid family that had come to include clinicians. This hybrid family had also been fraught with many conflicts and had changed over the years. To speak of Ronetta's life is very much to speak of life in the middle, of a life in suspense, one where family making of various kinds has constituted a crucial aspect of hope.

At the age of seventeen when we met up with her again, she looked back at those years in the hospital and the long process of recovery, a recovery not from the disease but from the worst ravages of the stroke itself. She recounted her horrifying awakening to a completely unfamiliar body and an alien world:

> I was in a coma for three days, and when I woke up, when I came out of the coma, I had memory loss. I didn't know where I was. I didn't remember anyone. I couldn't talk. I couldn't eat. I couldn't even move anymore.

Through intensive speech, occupational, and physical therapy, she learned "how to do everything all over again." The first time she was sent home from the hospital, she was still terribly disabled. "I couldn't eat and I couldn't walk," she said. "I could talk some and I was just learning to eat again but I had feeding tubes . . . I was even in diapers. Like I couldn't go to the restroom by myself," she recalled painfully.

Drawing primarily upon interviews with Ronetta and Ron (some conducted separately and some together), as well as Ron's discussions with us and other parents at the Collective Narrative Groups, I highlight three key events in Ronetta's life since the time of her stroke that reveal hope as a transformative journey, a hope that demanded she cultivate her skills and even self-identity as a "culture broker."

Recovering a Body and Creating a New Self

When we initially encountered Ronetta a few months after her stroke, she seemed utterly lost. She cried for her mother, she missed her father, she was in terrible pain, and she was very depressed. Ron, it will be remembered, feared that she had lost the will to live. Looking back, she admitted that she had been "pretty depressed" during that time. "It was discouraging . . . I would be like, I wish I could just pray and I'd walk again."

While walking, with its image of bodily repair, is present in Ronetta's account, walking as part of a transformative journey is much more vividly marked. It becomes embedded within a narrative of growing up, of cultivating a new kind of self, an increasingly more "independent" self. Her efforts to become a more self-sufficient person are connected to the exigencies of her family life and to her precarious medical status. This is not some triumphant narrative of American individualism but a transformative project born out of Ronetta's marginal status in clinical and family worlds.

Her father has never been too involved with her care, she has also noted more than once, and with evident sadness. She offers this evidence:

> If you asked him, like, what medications that I take, he couldn't tell you. If you asked him what kind of treatments do I receive, I guess he could tell you that I get transfusions. He knows that, but that's about it. If you asked him about sickle cell he couldn't tell you. Like, if he was a person on the street that you just asked about sickle cell, you wouldn't know that he has a child that has sickle cell because he couldn't tell you much of anything about it.

Though she is sure he loves her, she admits his lack of knowledge has been "pretty difficult."

> Sometimes that's kinda difficult for me because it seems like if you care about a person, especially something like that—your child having a disease—you would try to know all you can about it so that you could help your child. But he doesn't. He doesn't know anything really. And I know he loves me. That has nothing to do with his love for me. But it's kinda difficult. It's still pretty difficult.

Her response has been to learn to take care of herself, as much as possible:

> I've always had to know myself how to take care of myself because my dad, he never really took the time to learn. And my stepmother, Regina, she really could care less.

Initially, upon first returning from the hospital, she had to depend upon her stepmother to help her with medications and to provide care at home, a woman who, although she took responsibility, "could care less" about her. Ronetta's description of Regina did, indeed, seem apt. In those earlier years when Ronetta was in the hospital for so long, Ron had tried several times to get Regina to come to our Collective Narrative Groups. She finally did attend once but sat sternly in her chair, neither speaking nor smiling, as though she disapproved of the whole business. It was no surprise that she never returned.[2]

It is not difficult to imagine the trial it must have been for Ronetta to be so dependent upon Regina during a period of her life when she was summarily returned to infancy. Ronetta describes a growing determination in the face of Regina's indifference and her father's unwillingness to become intimately acquainted with her sickness and help with her care.

> I learned quickly how to take care of myself, like to be able to put on my own clothes, do my own feedings. What happened actually was I started to crawl around. You know how a baby does, like, before they know how to walk? I did that. I crawled around.

She crawled with a purpose, though, an angry determination. She crawled to become independent.

> Until I was able to walk again that's how I would get around the house . . . Because I felt like Regina, although she did do it, I felt like she didn't want to. And, like, my personality is, you don't have to help me if you don't want to. It'll get done. I'll make sure it gets done.

While during this period of hospitalizations many members of the clinical rehabilitation team complained that Ronetta kept returning "shaped like a chair," Ronetta has a different story to tell. She had three separate long hospitalizations over the two-year period, and she marks each of them as part of a path of progress. She remembers how depressed she was after the stroke. But she saw each of her hospitalizations and her growing independence from Regina as evidence of her victory in recovery. The second time she went into the hospital for a lengthy stay she relearned a whole new set of skills. She learned how to eat, how to talk again. "I was a lot better, but I was still in a wheelchair." The third stay marks what she labeled a full recovery where she learned to walk again:

> And then I went through therapy again for the third time. And that was the last time I went. And when I came home the third time I was fully recovered. I was walking again.

Creating a New "Hybrid Family"

One of the more remarkable examples of boundary crossing occurred a few months before Ronetta turned eighteen. She decided to move out of her father's house. Since she had never gotten on with her stepmother, even when she was much more physically independent, this had been a source of continued family tension throughout the years. A home health nurse who had known her since she was a child offered that she could come and live with her. And that is what Ronetta did. She came home to visit periodically. Her younger brother missed her tremendously, but her father seemed relieved. He liked this nurse who had become her godmother. She could finally get a mother's care, he told all of us at one of the Collective Narrative Groups after she had moved. "Now that she is eighteen, she really is a young lady and needs to make decisions on her own. Now my job is to focus on raising my son," he said. He has repeatedly shown pride in the maturity and rather remarkable school achievements of his daughter.

From Ronetta's point of view, these hard-won achievements have come not only because of her own efforts but especially because of how her home health nurse, Christine, came to play such a central role in her life. Christine had treated her for seven years, gradually assuming a double identity as both mother and nurse. Ronetta credits her with helping her to be able to achieve so well academically (staying consistently on the honor roll) even while she spent days and sometimes weeks in the hospital on a regular basis. She acknowledges how Christine became a "second mother" to her and how Christine's family became Ronetta's "godfamily."

> And like, her kids and her family, they're like a, a second family to me. I call them my godfamily. 'Cause they're like my, they're just like my family. We got really close and stuff and so she's like my godmother. And her kids are my godbrothers and sisters.

Home health nurses and aides are some of the most interesting border characters in clinical care. Many of those serving the families in this study are themselves African American, as Christine is. Many come from class backgrounds not so different from the families whose children they treat. They constitute the "working poor" more often than the middle class. When they develop close bonds with families, they may stay for many years. In such cases they often function as advocates, accompanying parents and children to clinical visits and to IEP (independent educational planning) meetings with school officials, functioning as mediators or sometimes just as moral support when a potentially hazardous and significant meeting or clinic visit is scheduled. They, more than hospital-based clinicians, often go well beyond the lines of official duties, becoming almost "adopted in" to some families. When the bonds are close, families often speak of them affectionately in kinship terms. ("She's my daughter's 'second mother,'{hrs}" they may say.) For parents with severely ill or disabled children who have become isolated because of the demand of caring for someone so medically fragile, these bonds can develop into some of the closest relationships they have.

Home health nurses are also some of the most hated and disrespected health professionals, from the families' perspective. Pay for this work is low, and many are not well trained or especially committed to their work. Some families have refused to hire them even when they could get the funding and badly needed the help, complaining that everyone they had hired was "lazy" and "neglectful." It is understandably difficult to find nurses that families can trust and feel safe to bring into their lives. Thus it says something both about Ronetta and her own home health nurse that they were able to forge such a close personal bond over the years.

Ronetta's move into Christine's house was a bit of an emergency rescue when, after a "huge argument" with her father, Ronetta decided to leave home though she did not have any good place to go. Christine took her in, initially, with the idea that she would stay only until she turned eighteen and could move into "Grove House," a house for young adults who had been in trouble or had little family. But when Ronetta did move into Grove House two months later, she "felt like it was unsafe."

> Some of the kids, I mean, you can imagine a place like that. The kids are trouble or whatever. And so there was kids fighting, doing drugs. I heard like some girls got raped there. And then also with my illness, I felt like I wasn't doing my best there, like as far as my health and stuff. So that's when I moved back with Christine.

For a while, all seemed to be going well with this new arrangement. But eventually it "came under stress," as Ronetta puts it, and she had to leave, returning back home. She tells, with some embarrassment and with prodding from both the researcher on the team (Kevin Groark) and her father, about a time when she got into trouble with Christine, admitting that perhaps she was putting too much "stress" on Christine by doing adolescent "dumb stuff." She gradually reveals the ways her behavior created tension with Christine. She also tries to underscore an empathic reading of Christine's mind, noting how she added to Christine's many burdens. Ronetta's very empathy suggests that while she had been so supported by her adopted "godfamily" she still had a marginal place in their lives. Her "adolescent dumb stuff" does, in fact, sound like the actions of a typical American teen, but Ronetta's tenuous status as a "god-daughter" did not entitle her to live within this family if she was going to behave in such troublesome adolescent ways. We also hear how her own health issues, and her failures to be compliant with her treatment regimen, formed a central part of Christine's complaints against her.

Ronetta: Yeah. But like the stress that I, that I guess I was putting on her [Christine], like me being a teen I would do dumb stuff or like . . .

Kevin: Can you give me an example of a dumb . . .

Ron: Doin' dumb stuff. What kinda dumb stuff?

Kevin: What's an example?

Ron: Yeah, that's what I'm waiting on.

Kevin: You can always say no if you don't wanna talk about it.

Ronetta: I'll talk about it. Like one night when I got drunk and like . . .

Kevin: Everybody's been there.

Ronetta: I threw up on her daughter's couch . . . I was in the bathroom and I fell backwards. Like, I was gettin' off the toilet or whatever and I bent forward and then I fell backwards into the shower. And I broke down the shower thing and stuff.

Kevin: How'd you get drunk? Were you by yourself? You got drunk by yourself or with friends?

Ronetta: No, I was at a party with her kids.

Kevin: Ohhh. Had you ever gotten drunk before?

Ronetta: No. But that's one example.

Kevin: She got really upset?

Ronetta: And like also because like over the years, like sometimes I don't take my medicine like I'm supposed to, like . . .

Kevin: Really? Still?

Ronetta: Yeah. Sometimes I don't because, not that I forget, I just, I just may not do it that day or something . . . Like I was supposed to like check my blood sugar and stuff. And like, I might miss a couple of days from checking the blood sugar or whatever because, like, I'll feel fine. I know when my sugar's high or when it's low or whatever. And she would get mad over things like that. Or even like me going out with my mom [Ronetta's biological mother] or something like that and being like kinda careless with my money . . .

Ron: Overspending or . . .

Ronetta: Maybe she would feel like I'm not doing anything around the house. Like she wanted me to do chores in the house, which, which I can understand, and like she might feel like I'm not doing enough or something like that. And it was like a lotta stress on her 'cause, like, by her husband's parents being sick, she didn't get to see him that much. Because he was always with them. And she was like kinda stressing over her husband and his health 'cause he's so worried about them, he's not taking care of his self. And she's also stressed over his parents being sick. And then her own kids have different stuff going on and she's like stressed over them. And her grandkids, also her friend had different things going on. She was thinking about them. And then she was having her own health problems and she's like stressed over her own health. And then she had *another case, another person that she was their nurse,* and the little girl and her mom would stress her out over their issues and stuff like that. So she had a lot on her plate.

Note that Ronetta's own "hybrid" status (as a child, a daughter but also a "case") is subtly marked in the last part of this passage. Referring to yet another person whose sickness was a burden to Christine, Ronetta refers to this child as "another case." Throughout Ronetta's interviews, Ronetta moves between identifiers when describing Christine. Sometimes she is a "nurse" (and by implication Ronetta is a "case"), and sometimes she is a mother.

Ronetta has come to see this period of life, and her return to her father's house, as another form of development. It is important to her that her father acknowledge she has matured. Again, she reframes even these embarrassing and difficult times in a genre of transformative journey, a journey that holds out the hope that she will one day be a clinician herself. Ron, too, feels he has changed through the course of their relationship and during the period when she moved away from the house. He remarks on his own past behavior in quite self-critical ways. His statements surprise and also gratify Ronetta. Both of them take advantage of the interviewing situation to open up to one another in ways that, it appears, they have not done before. Both explicitly mark the transformations that have occurred in their personal lives and in their relationship.

Ronetta: Yeah. I mean so far everybody's been getting along. I mean we have our moments and stuff, but we've been getting along so far. It's been pretty good.

Ron: I'd like to say something. That's one thing that I know I feel good about, that I'm able to understand her better now.

Ronetta: Thank you.

Kevin: Really?

Ron: Where I didn't take time off to really pay her much attention. When she get me to listen to her, or get a point across, I was only concerned about what I was thinking. But now since she had been away and come back, it's like we can communicate, you know, without, you know, bringing up something that's gonna come between what we're trying to establish. Because most of our understanding one another is through moral support. Because she's an adult now. I can't tell her what to do and how to do it and *(mimicking a stern fatherly voice)* "You shouldn't do it." And "Don't do it." So, all I'm really doing is trying to develop an understanding with her and love her like a father supposed to do his child. You know, and hope that she try and do better each day and take care of what she has to do. Because I can't do it for her no more. You know, and so far she's been holding up pretty good. On top at her school and all that stuff.

Kevin: So what's the change been like since when she was living with you before to now? How are things different?

Ronetta: Do you feel like I've matured?

Ron: I feel like she matured a lot. A great deal since before she left.

Hope and an Imagined Future Self: Ronetta Becomes the Clinician

Here we see a narrative developing in this family that constitutes both individual changes and relational, familial changes. In interviews conducted during the spring of 2009, Ronetta continued to speak of her dream to become a pediatric hematologist, one she was trying to realize through her education. She hoped to be able to transfer from community college in her junior year to UCLA. In these interviews, she offered a much more explicit account of her dream to "help other kids with sickle cell and blood disorders."

She was clear that her many years of experience with the disease had provided her with competencies and knowledge that had turned her into a kind of patient-clinician hybrid. "I have a really huge advantage," she contended, "because by me having sickle cell I know a lot about sickle cell and other diseases. Because I've been around the medical field all my life." This hybridity is wonderfully marked in the temporal ambiguity with which she described herself: "I feel like I'm my own doctor, though. *Although I'm not a doctor yet, I am a doctor.*" But her desire to become a hematologist stemmed from more than her familiarity with the disease. It was also about race and class. Like parents in the study whose children have sickle-cell anemia, and like many of the clinicians (white and black) who were on the sickle-cell team at her hospital, she noted its comparative neglect in race and class terms.

> I feel like sickle cell is looked over. Not a lot of people know about sickle cell. And it's not something that—like how cancer, how everyone is so concerned about getting a cure for cancer. And that's good and everything. We definitely need a cure for cancer. But sickle cell, we also need to be doing research on cures for sickle cell . . . I mean, it's mainly found in African American and like Pacific Islander and people of that origin. But it's a serious disease and like it needs to be known about. People need to know about it, and people need to be trying to find cures for that also.

She connected this societal neglect not only to race but to class. "It's found in African Americans, and in society, a lot of times, African Americans are like of the lower class." She paused, considering: "I don't know if in urban society, in society, the lower class doesn't count as much." She underscored—definitively this time—the reality of race and class in America. "So because it's found in more lower-class people it may be overlooked because they don't matter as much," she asserted matter-of-factly.

At the urging of her father, Ronetta disclosed her own painful humiliation and anger at being stigmatized by clinicians with essentially "ghetto" markers of street drug addiction. Although she felt trusted and well treated by the primary physicians whom she had known her whole life, when she went into the hospital with a pain crisis, residents and other physicians who did not know her often disbelieved that she was in any real pain.

> I feel like when I got to City Hospital for like my pain crisis and stuff that they don't wanna treat me because at City Hospital they say that I don't have any hemoglobin-S. And to them, that means that I can't have a pain crisis, when that's not true. Because sometimes I do still have a crisis. And I, and I get severe pain. And when I go there, they don't wanna treat me with the pain medicine and stuff that I may need at the moment. Like my direct doctors, like Dr. Heath and Dr. Morten and Dr. Williamson, they actually are good. It's actually the doctors like the residents . . . those doctors

are the ones I have problems with. They're the ones that actually treat me, treat me like I was saying—like they try to call me an addict and stuff. They're the ones that do that actually.

She told the following story in which her request for Benadryl to stop itching (a common side effect of medications) was reinterpreted by a physician as essentially a request for an illicit "ghetto" drug. She wanted it, he told her, because "this is like crack to you." She was highly offended by the obvious identification of a "street drug" with the commonly prescribed medication she had requested.

> Ronetta: And one doctor's like, because I have to take Benadryl with some of the medication 'cause it causes itching, and I'm supposed to get IV Benadryl with it, and they said, one of the doctors was like, "No you can't have IV Benadryl. We don't give IV Benadryl because it gives you a high. And the only reason you want it is because you like that high."
>
> Ron: *(in surprise)* They say that?
>
> Ronetta: Yeah. And that was the doctor—I told you—he was like, he came in there and he told me, "This is like crack to you. It's like crack cocaine. It gives you that type of high like that, and that's why you want it."
>
> Kevin: Wow.
>
> Ronetta: And I was like, "Excuse me. No. I'm supposed to have it because I have a reaction to this medication and it's to prevent the reaction."

Ronetta admitted that some of her friends or kids she knew from the sickle-cell clinic did fake a pain crisis to get high. She realized this was something clinicians were aware of, and she recognized that it was a problem for them. But still, she insisted, the clinicians were wrong, even morally wrong, to assign labels to her or anyone else as an automatic response. "Even so, they shouldn't generalize," she said repeatedly. It was wrong to "stereotype sickle-cell kids."

Finding a New Clinical Home

Her solution to this problem of labeling was ingenious. Unbeknownst to any clinicians at the City Hospital where she received all her "regular care" (meaning her transfusions) and where she would turn in a non-pain-related medical crisis, she had found another hospital just across the street where she went to be treated specifically for pain. She had done research on other hospitals that might be able to provide treatment. When she turned eighteen, she could be admitted as an adult, and she waited until that time to locate a hospital that she thought had experience in sickle-cell disease and might provide her better and more respectful care in managing her pain crises.

> That's why I decided to go to Cromwell Clinic. Well, I didn't off the bat choose Cromwell Clinic. Like I said, I did my research and stuff about it. But I had been planning to go to a different hospital because I was having, it seemed like every time I would go into the hospital I would have the same problem with the doctors like that. And they became increasingly disrespectful in that way, like trying to characterize me like an addict and just talking to me like I was ignorant and stupid . . . And it really made me angry . . . And so I went one day when I got real sick. I just I went there [to Cromwell Clinic]. I liked the hospital, I liked the doctors and their knowledge about my condition and stuff like that. So I felt comfortable there.

Becoming an effective culture broker in clinical worlds was critical to Ronetta's own journey. It demanded inventiveness as the course of an illness and life circumstances changed. She had become as adept as many of the parents not only in cultivating a stance of clinical authority over her disease (she was a doctor even though she was not yet a doctor) but also in making her way through the health care system. While she sometimes wanted to "go off" on the clinicians who had accused her of being a drug addict, she saw that she had to control herself. Instead, she cleverly developed a new set of clinical relationships at an entirely new hospital where she felt more "comfortable" and respected. She also kept connected to her former home health nurse and "godmother," continuing to work to mend the fractures that her stay in that household had created. And through her education she was trying to realize her hope of becoming the doctor she already, in one sense, was.

A (PROVISIONAL) ENDING

I might have ended this book in a different place, emphasizing the fleeting, precarious, or (more insidiously) governmental nature of institutionalized hope. Instead, I have chosen to return to the patients and families themselves for a final consideration of how hope is cultivated, practiced in everyday life. It has seemed important not to let the institutional (or the discursive) have the last word and instead to foreground how a "blues hope" is struggled for even by people with as few resources as Andrena and Ronetta.

In closing this book with Andrena and Ronetta, I have admittedly drawn upon two especially adept culture brokers. These are people who have endeavored in creative ways to cultivate new competencies and to revise the hopes that they have brought to their clinical relationships. By turning, in the end, to individual lives, extending a biographical gaze over a several-year period, I have also emphasized the person-centered nature of a narrative phenomenology of hope. Border crossing is a long-haul practice. It changes people. My stories of Andrena and Ronetta are not meant to advocate "blind optimism" or to promote some simple "romance of resistance" but to insist that if hope is to be discovered in all its vagaries, vulnerabilities, and paradoxes, one must look to personal and family lives. Notwithstanding the oppressive weight of dominating social orders or the durable routines of everyday life, we need dramatistic social theories in which persons are foregrounded in the midst of their plights and possibilities. Such persons are rarely clear-headed deliberators. They are inevitably muddled creatures buffeted by life's moral and practical complexities, confusions, mysteries, and obstacles. To end with their lives is to end in suspense, for it is still not clear what the future may bring.

Notes

1. THE LOBBY

1. For examples of considerations of this issue as part of the illness experience, see Becker (1994); Kleinman (1989); A. Frank (1995).

2. See also Reynolds (1989); G. Frank (2000); Morris (1998); Ingstad and Whyte (1995, 2007); Franklin (1997).

3. The issue of hope from the clinician's perspective has been addressed by M. Good et al. (1994) and in some of my own work (Mattingly 1994, 1998a).

4. I try to bring in this biographical dimension throughout the book in a number of ways. It is present in the design of this study, which has been carried out by following people (as Hollan [2001:55] suggests) "through time and space, and across different cultural domains." It is also present in the way I have chosen to analyze and represent the themes of this book. Through case studies that explore the meaning—the "at stakeness"—of particular moments to individual and family lives, I try to foreground this personal dimension of practice.

I offer portraits of individual lives (or, more accurately, bits of lives) and not merely typical social events or discursive formations partly to resist generalizations that transform people into cultural categories and types—into "familiar strangers." Person-centered writing offers a tactic for bringing those I write about closer to us, as readers and observers, rendering them "not as automatons programmed according to 'cultural' rules or acting out social roles, but as people going through life wondering what they should do" (Abu-Lughod 1993:27). Abu-Lughod describes this as a "tactical humanism," in which the plight of individuals is brought to the foreground. The individuals I speak about, like those Abu-Lughod presents, are "confronted with choices; they struggle with others, make conflicting statements, argue about points of view on the same events, undergo ups and downs in various relationships and changes in their circumstances and desires, face new pressures and fail to predict what will happen to them or those around them" (1993:14).

Writing in the language of particulars matters because even when one adopts apparently phenomenological theories and methods, they can lead as easily as anything else to typifications that ride roughshod over the personal. As Dorinne Kondo notes, the "liveliness and complexity of everyday life cannot be encompassed by theoretical models which rely on organizational structures, 'typical' individuals . . . or invocations of collective nouns" (1990:8). Instead of collective nouns and sui generis organizational structures, I try to portray the social world as a dwelling, as lived in, with all "its habituality, its crises, its vernacular and idiomatic character, its biographical particularities, its decisive events and indecisive strategies" (Jackson 1996:8).

5. See, for example, Jackson (1995, 2002); Olwig and Hastrup (1997); Clifford (1988, 1992, 1999); Appadurai (1986, 1991, 1996); Metcalf (2001); Paerregaard (1997), Meinert (2009).

6. Appadurai (1996); Bhabha (1994); Hyde (2008); Gupta and Ferguson (1997a).

7. This theme is nicely discussed by Browner and Preloran (2010) and is one I have also discussed in several earlier works (e.g., Mattingly 2003, 2006a, 2008a).

8. Elizabeth Traube (1996) notes the theoretical heritage of Gramsci in the current adoption of the "contested terrain" as the proper object of study.

9. See Fischer (2007) for a recent discussion of this.

10. Violent acts based upon racial markers are also naming acts, acts of language. "There's no racism without a language. The point is not that acts of racial violence are only words but rather that they have to have a word. Even though it offers the excuse of blood, color, birth—or rather, because it uses this naturalist and sometimes creationist discourse—racism always betrays the perversion of a man, the 'talking animal.' It institutes, declares, writes, inscribes, prescribes. A system of marks, it outlines space in order to assign forced residence or to close off borders. It does not discern, it discriminates" (Derrida 1985:331).

11. This insistence is also evident in clinical work. Clinicians may object that their patients push them for "the numbers," which they saw as "undercutting hope" (M. Good et al. 1990:98).

12. Obama seemed to call regularly upon this hope in his own campaign speeches as when, during the New Hampshire primaries, he countered Hilary Clinton's accusation that he was promoting "false hope" with these words: "We've been asked to pause for a reality check. We've been warned against offering the people of this nation false hope. But in the unlikely story that is America, there has never been anything false about hope" (Obama, quoted in Miyazaki 2008:5). Journalists have continued to marvel at Obama's enormous popularity and "the remarkable surge of hope in an otherwise downbeat, if not depressing, period" (Herbert 2009:A1).

13. In the months after the election, journalists, bloggers, and television commentators echoed these words since Obama rose to prominence: "We need to send a message to ourselves and to the world that we truly do stand for life, liberty and the pursuit of happiness. And in electing an African-American, we also profoundly renounce an ugliness and violence in our national character

that have been further stoked by our president in these last eight years" (Wenner 2008).

14. There is an even more complicated story to tell because several studies that have looked at the relationships between African American clinicians and African American patients argue that issues of trust are not significantly less problematic, a topic I take up in chapter 3.

2. NARRATIVE MATTERS

1. Some social theorists have worked to bring Marx into contemporary practice theory through the development of "activity theory" (e.g., Chaiklin and Lave 1996). Closely related is a cultural-historical tradition of practice theory especially inspired by the work of Lev Vygotsky that has influenced cognitive and educational anthropologists as well as cultural psychologists (Lave and Wenger 1991; Lave 1988; Holland et al. 1998; Dreier 2008; Wertsch 2002; Hedegaard and Fleer 2008).

2. Some texts that have addressed this issue include V. Turner and Bruner (1986); Throop (2010, 2003); Desjarlais (1997); Kleinman and Kleinman (1991); Mattingly (1998a, 2000); Biehl, Good, and Kleinman (2007).

3. As Kleinman, Das, and Lock put it: "The trauma, pain, and disorders to which atrocity gives rise are health conditions; yet they are also political and cultural matters. Similarly, poverty is the major risk factor for ill health and death; yet this is only another way of saying that health is a social indicator and indeed a social process" (1997: ix). Beyond the general concern to bring together the structural and the experiential, three developments within this line of work bear close connection to the narrative phenomenology of practice I will outline. First, they share an emphasis upon social and political borderlands, spaces that are not primarily geographical ones but inhabited, embodied ones, existing in and through the subjectivities of people (Hyde 2008:192). Second, attention to smaller, more intimate social units (like the family) also serves as a means to challenge and complicate analytic polarizations between the individual on the one hand and nation or social institution on the other, polarizations that have also contributed to a false dichotomy between experience and structure (Gordon and Paci 1997; Eaton 2008). Finally there is a focus not only on suffering but also on healing as both an individual matter and a matter connected to the healing of community, the struggle to "remake a world" (Das et al. 2001). Here, especially, "hope" emerges as a central aspect of the experience of suffering.

4. On narrative in relation to the temporality of lived experience, see Ricoeur (1984, 1985), Carr (1991), Olafson (1979), and V. Turner (1969, 1986b); in relation to the self, see MacIntyre (1981); Taylor (1989), and Ricoeur (1984, 1985, 1988); in relation to moral action and ethics, see MacIntyre (1981) and Taylor (1989); in relation to suffering, see Kleinman (1989), Hydén and Brockmeier (2008), and Mishler (1986), as well as Garro and Mattingly (2000), for an extended literature review on the role of narrative in studies of suffering and healing; and in relation to the structure of thought, see J. Bruner (1986, 1990).

5. For example, Wertsch (2002); Holland et al. (1998).

6. I have learned especially from a few thinkers whose works have inspired me over the years: Kenneth Burke, Victor Turner, Jerome Bruner, Alisdair MacIntyre, Charles Taylor, Paul Ricoeur, David Carr, Clifford Geertz, Hans-Georg Gadamer, and Wolfgang Iser.

7. In making such claims, I am drawing upon the hermeneutic phenomenology of Heidegger, Gadamer, Ricoeur, and Carr, who stress that experience is not purely personal and cannot ever be purely immediate; in fact, they insist, it is deeply rooted in the sociality of historical experience.

8. Gadamer critiques Dilthey for his inability to adequately credit the powerful role of the socially shared in building his concept of understanding. For Gadamer, Dilthey offers an overly personal, even biographical notion of the hermeneutic experience: "Self-reflection and autobiography—Dilthey's starting-points—are not primary and are not an adequate basis for the hermeneutical problem, because through them history is made private once more. In fact history does not belong to us, but we belong to it. Long before we understand ourselves through the process of self-examination, we understand ourselves in a self-evident way in the family, society and state in which we live. The focus of subjectivity is a distorting mirror" (Gadamer 1975:245).

While recognizing the importance of Gadamer's argument, my own version of hermeneutic phenomenology preserves something from Dilthey that I believe that Gadamer and Ricoeur lost sight of. We might, as individuals, arrive with our history in hand, so to speak, but I am unwilling to go as far as Gadamer, who remarks: "The self-awareness of the individual is only a flickering in the closed circuits of historical life" (1975:245). Or again, "The anticipation of meaning that governs our understanding of a text is not an act of subjectivity, but proceeds from the communality that binds us to the tradition. But this is contained in our relation to tradition, in the constant process of education. Tradition is not simply a precondition into which we come, but we produce it ourselves, inasmuch as we understand, participate in the evolution of tradition and hence further determine it ourselves" (1975:261).

In this narrative phenomenology I depart from Gadamer in some respects, for I am unwilling to accept his wholesale rejection of the "romantic" hermeneutics that advocated some method of personal empathy as part of the path toward understanding. This Diltheyian hermeneutics kept alive the subjectivity of understanding. The critique Gadamer (and Heidegger before him) made of this was that it kept alive precisely a metaphysics that they sought to go beyond. Gadamer accused Dilthey of still being caught in an Enlightenment epistemology that insisted on a separation of subject and object. Gadamer rejected any version of this. That is, he rejected the idea of a subject who, through the practice of some correct method, can know things as they truly are (an idea inherent in Cartesian subject/object epistemology).

9. This is not to say that we simply live out stories. There is an undoubted difference between life as lived and life as narrated through stories, as many commentators have pointed out. Whatever else we can say, life as lived cannot be equated with life as narrated, many would strongly contend (e.g., E. Bruner 1986; R. Bauman 1986; Jackson 2002). Narrative is commonly viewed as a textual activity that does "narrative violence" (in Ricouer's [1984] felicitous

phrase) to experience in the very attempt to render it into words. The violence may be for literary effect or, reflecting a predominant anthropological view, may express a human need for meaning, the quest to render the unsayable, the inchoate, into some kind of coherent cultural form. But, to echo a response I have made before (Mattingly 1998a, 2000), I do not think life as lived is as incoherent as some presume, or that stories—as texts—are as coherent and unitary. More to the point, I do not think a notion of coherence and unity is primarily what narrative has to offer to social theory. Ricoeur offers an intriguing suggestion about why this idea of experience as incoherent and unsayable has been so compelling for contemporary scholars of the last several decades: "We ought to ask . . . whether the plea for a radically unformed temporal experience is not itself the product of a fascination for the unformed that is one of the features of modernity" (1984:72).

10. See Park's (2008) exquisite analysis of a clinical encounter as an illustration of this principle.

11. Preunderstanding also involves prejudging. This is a picture of knowledge that Enlightenment thinkers were especially concerned to deny in their attempt to ground knowledge in an objective, ahistorical, and unsituated mind. "It is not until the enlightenment that the concept of prejudice acquires the negative aspect we are familiar with. Actually 'prejudice' means a judgment that is given before all the elements that determine a situation have been finally examined" (Gadamer 1975:239–40). Notably, the conception of experience and its relationship to preunderstanding as developed in hermeneutic phenomenology is very distinct from Husserl's notion of "bracketing."

12. Within phenomenological hermeneutics, distinctions are made between "an experience" or "significant experience" versus "mere experience" in a way that I call upon in my own work (e.g., Gadamer 1975).

13. This has been an insight developed by a number of linguistic anthropologists (e.g., Ochs and Capps 2001). See also Arthur Frank (2010) and Catherine Riessman (2008) for readable and highly insightful treatments of this perspective.

14. A wealth of writing examines this across several disciplines, including sociolinguistics, linguistic anthropology, and folklore theory. Some particularly seminal and useful texts are E. Bruner (1984, 1986); E. Bruner and Gorfain (1984); and R. Bauman (1986). Mishler (1986) also provides some classic work on storytelling (and its suppression) within the clinical encounter.

15. In a later chapter, I will explore how children (with the cooperation of parents) identify with Disney and other fantasy narratives, drawing upon this as a form of play. This playing with stories is beautifully described by Ricoeur as a kind of proposal that the narrative offers its audience. As part of our reception of the story, we are following, not words, but something much subtler and more imaginative—the text proposes "a world that I might inhabit." Interpreting the story is, in fact, just this act of "proposing of a world that I might inhabit and into which I might project my ownmost powers" (1984:81).

16. Arthur Frank (1995) has offered a particularly insightful analysis of some overarching, culturally shaped narrative genres of healing. Though his genres do not match mine precisely, two are particularly salient for my purposes.

One he calls a "restitution narrative," a canonical medical genre that relies on the idea of body as machine. The restitution genre speaks to a plot structure deeply implicated in the cultural project of biomedicine and its telos, its practical hope: the cure. This genre is our "culturally preferred narrative," one that is so compelling because it seems to "exorcise" mortality itself by "deconstructing it" (1995:83–84). He also identifies a second genre, healing as a quest, which I take up in my discussion of healing as "transformative journey."

17. As M. J. Good puts it: "The affective and imaginative dimensions of biomedicine and biotechnology envelop physicians, patients and the public in a 'biotechnical embrace'" (2007:364).

18. Many anthropological commentators have also used biomedicine as a case study for viewing Western rationality's claims to universality and objectivity as a false hope (Casper and Koenig 1996; Comaroff 1982; Foucault 1973, 1979; B. Good 1994; Lock and Gordon 1988; Taussig 1980). They have offered cogent critiques of Enlightenment ideals of truth, rationality, and progress that have undergirded Western biomedicine and its specious claims to universal truth.

Anthropologists have carried out global ethnographic explorations of how the dream of better health and the possibilities of progress based on medical science have provided new opportunities for control of the sick, who, with their own personal hopes for care and cure, are transformed into new kinds of political subjects willing to undergo new kinds of subjugation. One dominant argument is that when illness is treated, as in canonical biomedicine, as something that belongs to an individual, political and social factors that have created the conditions for its possibility are disguised. Lock points out, "In North America particularly, efforts to reduce suffering have habitually focused on control and repair of individual bodies. The social origins of suffering and distress, including poverty and discrimination, even if fleetingly recognized, are set aside, while effort is expended in controlling disease and averting death through biomedical manipulations" (1997:210). Farmer has made a very strong case for how this has happened with infectious diseases. Speaking of tuberculosis, he writes, "We cannot understand its markedly patterned occurrence—in the United States, for example, afflicting those in homeless shelters and in prison—without understanding how social forces, ranging from political violence to racism, come to be embodied as individual pathology. . . . Thus do fundamentally social forces and processes come to be embodied as biological events" (1999:13–14).

Health easily becomes, as Veena Das puts it, a "contested site," even a site "for the exercise of new kinds of power" over the suffering in the name of offering medical help (1994:163). The kind of coercion that medicine exerts is very often a subtle kind. New opportunities for health care—new practices—help to shape people's hopes, and these hopes may, in turn, betray them. Nancy Scheper-Hughes offers an example from her research in Brazil, where the poor receive "treatment" for disease conditions that should properly be reframed in economic and political terms. The essential economic basis of their hunger becomes "medicalized" as a nervous condition that should be responded to with tranquilizers and the like. She speaks of this as a "glaring example . . . of the misuse of medical knowledge" (1993:170). Her analysis, drawing from both Gramsci and Foucault, is directed especially to the role of the expert doctor in maintaining this fiction of individual illness in the midst of overwhelmingly obvious poverty. To make matters worse, because medicine operates with an emphasis on the patient as location of disease, patients are often blamed for the diseases that afflict them.

19. The rise of new biotechnologies has greatly expanded this genre. Clinicians are now able to detect the possibility of disease prior to its occurrence, as when genetic testing allows individuals to assess the risks of having children in light of their own genetic makeup. This technology instills new hope for families and clinicians by offering the potential for preventative treatment in those predicted to develop certain diseases or for detecting potential problems of disease manifestation before they happen. For example, a clinician in our study talks about recent research on sickle-cell disease that may offer the possibility of "predicting who's gonna have more problems," thereby allowing clinicians to watch patients more closely and offer more aggressive treatment.

20. The successful patient may be depicted as the "victor" or "survivor" of the fight. When the body does not mobilize sufficiently to defeat the enemy, very ill or dying patients often come to experience their bodies as *overtaken* by illness, feeling that they have lost the battle with disease (Lawton 2000:77). M. Good et al. (1990) and Gordon (1990), however, complicate this picture. They argue that the image of cancer is gradually changing from death, hopelessness, and "condemned" "victims" to a heroic metaphor of "survivors" (Mullan 1985), "victors" (Pepper 1984), or "exceptional patients" (Siegel 1993). According to M. Good et al. (1990), cancer patients now may confront cancer through a "discourse of hope," as a challenge that can be "beat" with a "fighting spirit" (quoted in Weiss 1997:458).

21. An excellent example concerns the promises of stem cell research to provide unprecedented means for tackling severe or even fatal diseases. "A direct media feeder system links developments in stem cell research to the possibility of treatment for severe, disabling, and often fatal conditions—binding stem cell technology securely into a rhetorical fabric of hope, health, and an improved future through increasing biological control" (Franklin 2005:59). Even nations can tell stories about themselves based on this promise. They can figure as the heroic healers, the new warriors who have come to the fore in an ancient battle—the war against disease. Franklin illustrates: "The United Kingdom is currently the 'world leader' in stem cell technologies. As Business Week reported in April of 2002, 'In stem cell research, it's rule Britannia'" (2005:59).

22. Arthur Frank offers a telling example. "A Nobel prize-winning physician was interviewed in my morning paper. He suggested that for the reporter to understand his work, he should think of the body as a television set." Frank goes on to comment: "The mechanistic view normalizes the illness: televisions break and require fixing, and so do bodies" (1995:88).

23. This is a narrative genre that "meet(s) suffering head on. . . . Illness is the occasion of a journey that becomes a quest. What is quested for may never

be wholly clear, but the quest is defined by the ill person's belief that something is to be gained through the experience" (A. Frank 1995:115). This narrative genre very clearly marks healing as a task that must be undertaken by the afflicted themselves. Frank offers a plot structure in three parts: departure (triggered by a symptom), an initiation ("the road of trials" [1995:118]), and a return (a resolution that is always in some way unalterably marked by the illness). Drawing on my own ethnographic work, I make this plot structure more subjunctive and with less resolution. There are, at best, certain moments that offer a "sense of an ending," potential resting places in what turns out to be an unending "road of trials." This road, precisely because it has no stopping point (at least not in this world), demands an apparently endless task of personal transformation.

24. It sometimes involves a call to become a "wounded healer." This is a culturally compelling figure in an array of cultures (Davis Floyd and St. John 1998; Laderman 1996), one that, within Western traditions, also has ancient roots in both religious and secular mythology.

25. It has also been enunciated by a host of scholars writing in the 1980s who have a clinical background (e.g., Mishler 1986; Kleinman 1989; Brody 1987; Coles 1988). Speaking from other clinical disciplines, this perspective has also been eloquently elaborated by such key clinical figures as Oliver Sacks (1984, 1987, 1995) and Luria (1987), who not only are magnificent storytellers in their own right but argue the need to understand their patients' illnesses narratively and attend to the stories that patients themselves tell.

Psychotherapeutic clinical disciplines like psychiatry, clinical psychology, clinical social work, and psychoanalysis have historically relied heavily upon narrative as part of their "talking cure." They have presumed that treatment involves treating the illness in biographical and narrative terms. While the specifically narrative character of the psychotherapeutic disciplines has not always been attended to, beginning in the 1980s several influential scholars explicitly focused on the centrality of narrative in these treatment traditions (e.g., Spence 1982; Young 1995; Schafer 1981, 1992; Capps and Ochs 1995a, 1995b; Waitzkin and Magana 1997). More recently, Tanya Luhrmann (2000) has looked at the schism that has grown up within psychiatry between an older and dominant narrative-based practice and a more recent and fundamentally biological one in which drugs rather than storytelling are the primary avenue for cure. What is important here is not simply that storytelling is part of the practice but that healing itself comes to be connected to a paradigmatically different perspective, one that connects illness and healing to the idea of personal transformation.

26. Rita Charon, in the United States, and Trisha Greenhalgh and Brian Hurwitz, in the United Kingdom, are the vanguard of this movement. It has arisen as a protest against the reductionism and biologism of contemporary medical care and has been inspired by some of the scholars I noted earlier and by the development of "narrative ethics." In one sense it is a kind of protest movement against medicine's canonical plots, not in the sense that they are necessarily wrong, but in the sense that they leave out so much of what is at stake for patients.

There is very often an insistence on the personalness, the singularity, of the illness experience. What is needed is to "reconcile the subjectivity and uniqueness of human experience with the physical reality of the body and a larger impersonal picture" (Hurwitz, Greenhalgh, and Skultans 2004:3). The claim here is that illness is an experience in which healing involves some sort of personal transformation and that narrative is important to it. Medicine, so the argument goes, should not only attend to the biographical disruption that can accompany illness but support, even guide, the work of personal transformation that illness calls for. Advocates of narrative medicine work to train clinicians to both listen to and tell stories, treating this skill as an integral aspect of the clinician's craft. In an article in the prestigious (and highly canonical) *Journal of the American Medical Association,* Charon argues that physicians need "narrative competence, that is, the competence that human beings use to absorb, interpret, and respond to stories" (2001:1897). Such competence, she further suggests, "enables the physician to practice medicine with empathy, reflection, professionalism, and trustworthiness" (1897).

At the heart of this movement is also an ethical ideal. The moral is brought back into clinical practice in a central way: the idea that the ethics of care are essential, that a "narrative ethics" ought to inform clinical practice in a much more fundamental way than the canonical vision of clinical practice allows, and that this perspective reveals "the particularities of individuals, the singularity of beliefs, the perspectival nature of truth, and the duties of intersubjectivity" (Charon 2004:27).

3. BORDER TROUBLE

1. Doescher et al. (2000); Lillie-Blanton et al. (2000); R. Johnson et al. (2004); LaVeist, Nickerson, and Bowie (2000).

2. Cooper-Patrick et al. (1999); M. Good et al. (2002); van Ryn and Burke (2000); van Ryn and Fu (2003).

3. Stone (2002); Canto et al. (2000); Hannan et al. (1999); Chin, Zhang, and Merrell (1998); Todd et al. (2000); Segal, Bola, and Watson (1996).

4. Whitehead (1997); Bailey (1991).

5. A concise article that details this can be found in van Ryn and Burke (2000).

6. In this section I have drawn extensively on Brodenheimer and Grumbach's (2002) excellent discussion of the health care delivery system in the United States. Unless otherwise noted, statistics are from this source. The figures provided here may change once again through the influence of health care reform legislation that has recently been introduced—as of spring 2010. It is too soon to tell how broadly these reforms will influence the general trends of health care delivery, the education of health practitioners, or the specific impact on African Americans.

7. It should be remembered that one of the highly troublesome features of health care delivery in the United States is that people with little or no health insurance who lack primary physicians often must rely upon emergency rooms for routine medical care. Since African Americans have significantly less health

insurance and are significantly more impoverished than their white counter-parts, they are part of the demographic comparatively more likely to end up in emergency rooms for such routine problems. Thus it is not hard to imagine how Andrena's racial status might have influenced her dismissal by a harried emergency room physician.

4. WIDENING THE GAP

1. As noted earlier, enlightenment thinkers were especially concerned to ground knowledge in an objective, ahistorical mind. This concern gave prejudice its bad name. To quote Gadamer once more: "It is not until the Enlightenment that the concept of prejudice acquires the negative aspect we are familiar with. Actually 'prejudice' means a judgment that is given before all the elements that determine a situation have been finally examined" (1975:239–40).

2. See Bruns (1992), Gadamer (2004), and Thompson (1984) for good discussions of the hermeneutic portrait of understanding as an encounter with otherness that ideally results in a subsequent "widening of horizons."

5. PLOTTING HOPE

1 . See Laderman and Roseman (1996) and V. Turner and Bruner (1986) for two seminal collections of essays on the aesthetics and performative qualities of social action and experience.

2. There is a rich literature on this subject within anthropology. Some influ-ential texts that have played a primary role in developing this phenomenological tradition within recent decades include Jackson (1989); Schieffelin (1996, 1998); Briggs (1996); Csordas (1994, 1995, 1996); Tambiah (1985); Laderman (1996); Stoller (1989, 1996, 1997); Hughes-Freeland (1998); Kapferer (1983, 1986); Schechner (1990); Danforth (1989); V. Turner (1969, 1986a, 1986b); E. Turner (1992); Desjarlais (1997); and Mattingly (1998a, 2004).

3. See Mattingly and Lawlor (2001); Mattingly (1998a).

6. DAYDREAMING

1. For examples of this globalized cultural inventiveness in a variety of societal contexts, see Abu-Lughod (1991); Appadurai (1991); Metcalf (2001); Diouf (2000); Mbembe (1992); Pollock et al. (2000); Price (1999); Erlmann (1996); Schein (2002); Mattingly (2003, 2006a).

2. This example comes from Stephanie Mielke, an experienced clinician who told this story in a class I was teaching.

3. Metcalf (2001); Abu-Lughod (1991); Appadurai (1991).

4. Spitulnik (1993); Caughie (1981, 1984); de Certeau (1984); Hebdige (1988).

5. This is a perspective voiced, for example, by Ernst Bloch, whose discus-sion of hope I have found, in other respects, so compelling and useful. Though Bloch spoke of film as a powerful new "dream factory" in the production of genuine and emancipatory hope, he held an especially scathing view of Ameri-

can cinema as offering only "rotten" dreams. "Thanks to America," he declared, "the film has become the most desecrated form of art" (1986:410).

6. Notably, throughout the Caribbean, as in several other parts of the world, a number of folktales feature mermaids.

7. FLEETING HOPE

1. B. Good (1994); Hahn and Gaines (1985:11).

2. Becker and Kaufman (1995); Rhodes (1995).

3. Browner and Preloran (2010); Lock (1996).

4. This example is taken from research that Mary Lawlor and I conducted in Chicago just prior to the Los Angeles study; it illustrated to both of us how precarious healing moments can be. Returning to this clinical case over the years has inspired me to reconsider the clinician-patient partnership and the centrality of hope in forging that bond.

5. Rhodes (1995); Petersen (2003); J. Powell and Biggs (2004).

6. Mattingly and Lawlor (2003); Mattingly and Fleming (1994).

7. On Western biomedicine's undermining of confidence in the embodied knowledge of sufferers, see Browner and Press (1995); Sargent and Bascope (1996).

8. NARRATIVE PHENOMENOLOGY AND THE PRACTICE OF HOPE

1. For example, innovations in biotechnology and their democratizing possibilities (Haraway 1997, Rose 2007).

2. Regina did come to the Collective Narrative family reunion that we held in April 2010 because of some dramatic changes in the family. However, it is beyond the scope of this book to document this unfolding story.

References

Abu-Lughod, Lila. 1991. "Writing against Culture." In *Recapturing Anthropology: Working in the Present*, edited by Richard G. Fox, 137–62. Santa Fe, NM: School of American Research Press.

———. 1993. *Writing Women's Worlds: Bedouin Stories*. Berkeley: University of California Press.

———. 2008. "Culture and Women's Rights: The Challenge of the Particular: A New Preface for the Twenty-first Century, L.A." In *Writing Women's Worlds: Bedouin Stories*, 2nd ed., edited by Lila Abu-Lughod, xi–xviii. Berkeley: University of California Press.

American Federation of Labor and Congress of Industrial Organizations. 2006. "Fast Facts: African Americans (2006)." www.aflcio.org/issues/civilrights/upload/africanamerican.pdf.

Amsterdam, Anthony G., and Jerome Bruner. 2000. *Minding the Law*. Cambridge, MA: Harvard University Press.

Appadurai, Arjun, ed. 1986. *The Social Life of Things: Commodities in Cultural Perspective*. Cambridge: Cambridge University Press.

———. 1991. "Global Ethnoscapes: Notes and Queries for a Transnational Anthropology." In *Interventions: Anthropologies of the Present*, edited by Richard G. Fox, 191–210. Santa Fe, NM: School of American Research.

———. 1996. *Modernity at Large: Cultural Dimensions of Globalization*. Minneapolis: University of Minnesota Press.

Appiah, K. Anthony, and Amy Gutmann. 1996. *Color Conscious: The Political Morality of Race*. Princeton: Princeton University Press.

Aristotle. 1967. *Poetics*. Translated by Gerald Frank Else. Ann Arbor: University of Michigan Press.

Atwater, Deborah F. 2007. "Senator Barack Obama: The Rhetoric of Hope and the American Dream." *Journal of Black Studies* 38 (2): 121–29.

Bailey, Eric J. 1991. "Hypertension: An Analysis of Detroit African-American Health Care Treatment Patterns." *Human Organization* 50 (3): 287–96.

Bauman, Richard. 1986. *Story, Performance and Event: Contextual Studies of Oral Narrative.* Cambridge: Cambridge University Press.

Bauman, Zygmunt. 1999. *Culture as Praxis.* Thousand Oaks, CA: Sage Publications.

Becker, Gay. 1994. "Metaphors in Disrupted Lives: Infertility and Cultural Constructions of Continuity." *Medical Anthropology Quarterly* 8:383–410.

Becker, G.K., and S.R. Kaufman. 1995. "Managing an Uncertain Illness Trajectory in Old Age: Patients' and Physicians' Views of Stroke." *Medical Anthropology Quarterly* 9 (2): 165–87.

Bhabha, Homi. 1994. *The Location of Culture.* New York: Routledge.

Biehl, João, Byron Good, and Arthur Kleinman, eds. 2007. *Subjectivity: Ethnographic Investigations.* Berkeley: University of California Press.

Bloch, Ernst. 1986. *The Principle of Hope.* Vol. 1. Translated by Neville Plaice, Stephen Plaice, and Paul Knight. Cambridge, MA: MIT Press.

Bluebond-Langner, Myra. 1996. *In the Shadow of Illness: Parents and Siblings of the Chronically Ill Child.* Princeton: Princeton University Press.

Bourdieu, Pierre. 1977. *Outline of a Theory of Practice.* Translated by Richard Nice. Cambridge: Cambridge University Press.

———. 1980. *The Logic of Practice.* Stanford: Stanford University Press.

———. 1987. *In Other Words: Essays towards a Reflexive Sociology.* Translated by Matthew Anderson. Stanford: Stanford University Press.

Bourdieu, Pierre, and Loïc Wacquant. 1992. *An Invitation to Reflexive Sociology.* Chicago: University of Chicago Press.

Briggs, Charles L. 1996. "The Meaning of Nonsense, the Poetics of Embodiment, and the Production of Power in Warao Healing." In *The Performance of Healing,* edited by Carol Laderman and Marina Roseman, pp. 185–232. London: Routledge.

Brodenheimer, Thomas S., and Kevin Grumbach. 2002. *Understanding Health Policy: A Clinical Approach.* 3rd ed. New York: McGraw-Hill Medical.

Brody, Howard. 1987. *Stories of Sickness.* New Haven: Yale University Press.

Browner, C.H., and N.A. Press. 1995. "The Normalization of Prenatal Diagnostic Screening." In *Conceiving the New World Order: The Politics of Reproduction,* edited by Faye D. Ginsburg and Rayna Rapp, pp. 307–22. Berkeley: University of California Press.

Browner, C.H., and M. Preloran. 2010. *Neurogenetic Diagnoses.* New York: Routledge.

Bruner, Edward M. 1984. "Introduction: The Opening Up of Anthropology." In *Text, Play and Story: The Construction and Reconstruction of Self and Society,*, edited by Edward M. Bruner, 1–16. Prospect, IL: Waveland Press.

———. 1986. "Ethnography as Narrative." In *The Anthropology of Experience,* edited by Victor W. Turner and Edward M. Bruner, 139–58. Urbana: University of Illinois Press.

Bruner, Edward M., and P. Gorfain. 1984. "Dialogic Narration and the Paradoxes of Masada." In *Text, Play and Story,* edited by Edward M. Bruner, 56–79. Prospect, IL: Waveland Press.

Bruner, Jerome. 1986. *Actual Minds, Possible Worlds.* Cambridge, MA: Harvard University Press.

———. 1990. *Acts of Meaning.* Cambridge, MA: Harvard University Press.

Bruns, Gerald L. 1992. *Hermeneutics Ancient and Modern.* New Haven: Yale University Press.

Bunche, Lonnie G., III. 1990. "A Past Not Necessarily Prologue." In *Twentieth Century Los Angeles: Power, Promotion, and Social Conflict,* edited by Norman M. Klein and Martin S. Shiesl, 101–30. Claremont, CA: Regina Books.

Burke, Kenneth. 1945. *A Grammar of Motives.* Berkeley: University of California Press.

———. 1966. *Language as Symbolic Action: Essays on Life, Literature, and Method.* Berkeley: University of California Press.

Canto, J. G., J. J. Allison, C. I. Kiefe, C. Fincher, R. Farmer, P. Sekar, S. Person, et al. 2000. "Relation of Race and Sex to the Use of Reperfusion Therapy in Medicare Beneficiaries with Acute Myocardial Infarction." *New England Journal of Medicine* 342 (15): 1094–1100.

Capps, Lisa, and Elinor Ochs. 1995a. *Constructing Panic: The Discourse of Agoraphobia.* Cambridge: Cambridge University Press.

———. 1995b. "Out of Place: Narrative Insights into Agoraphobia." *Discourse Process* 19:407–40.

Carr, David. 1991. *Time, Narrative, and History.* Bloomington: Indiana University Press.

Casper, M. J., and B. A. Koenig. 1996. "Reconfiguring Nature and Culture: Intersections of Medical Anthropology and Technoscience Studies." *Medical Anthropology Quarterly* 10 (4): 523–36.

Cassel, Joan. 1991. *Expected Miracles: Surgeons at Work.* Philadelphia: Temple University Press.

Caughie, John. 1981. "Progressive Television and Documentary Drama." In *Popular Television and Film: A Reader,* edited by Tony Bennett, Susan Boyd-Bowman, Colin Mercer, and Janet Woollacott, 327–52. London: British Film Institute.

———. 1984. "Television Criticism: 'A Discourse in Search of an Object.'" *Screen* 25 (4–5): 109–20.

Chaiklin, Seth, and Jean Lave, eds. 1996. *Understanding Practice: Perspectives on Activity and Context.* Cambridge: Cambridge University Press.

Charon, Rita. 2001. "Narrative Medicine: A Model for Empathy, Reflection, Profession, and Trust." *Journal of the American Medical Association* 286:1897–1902.

———. 2004. "The Ethicality of Narrative Medicine." In *Narrative Research in Health and Illness,* edited by Brian Hurwitz, Trisha Greenhalgh, and Vieda Skultans, 23–36. Oxford: Blackwell.

———. 2006. *Narrative Medicine: Honoring the Stories of Illness.* Oxford: Oxford University Press.

Chin, M. H., J. X. Zhang, and K. Merrell. 1998. "Diabetes in the African-American Medicare Population: Morbidity, Quality of Care, and Resource Utilization." *Diabetes Care* 21:1090–95.

Clifford, James. 1988. *The Predicament of Culture: Twentieth-Century Ethnography, Literature, and Art.* Cambridge, MA: Harvard University Press.

———. 1992. "Traveling Cultures." In *Cultural Studies,* edited by Larry Grossberg, Cary Nelson, and Paula Treichler, 96–116. London: Routledge.

———. 1997. *Routes: Travel and Translation in the Twentieth Century.* Cambridge, MA: Harvard University Press.

———. 1999. "After Writing Culture: Review Essay." *American Anthropologist* 101 (3): 643–46.

Coles, Robert. 1988. *The Call of Stories: Teaching and Moral Imagination.* Cambridge, MA: Harvard University Press.

Comaroff, Jean. 1982. "Medicine: Symbol and Ideology." In *The Problem of Medical Knowledge: Examining the Social Construction of Medicine,* edited by Peter Wright and Andrew Treacher, 49–57. Edinburgh: Edinburgh University Press.

Cooper-Patrick, L., J. Gallo, J. Gonzales, H. Vu, N. Powe, C. Nelson, and D. Ford. 1999. "Race, Gender, and Partnership in the Patient-Physician Relationship." *Journal of the American Medical Association* 282 (6): 583–89.

Crapanzano, Vincent. 2004. *Imaginative Horizons: An Essay in Literary-Philosophical Anthropology.* Chicago: University of Chicago Press.

Csordas, Thomas J. 1994. *The Sacred Self: A Cultural Phenomenology of Charismatic Healing.* Berkeley: University of California Press.

———, ed. 1995. *Embodiment and Experience: The Existential Ground of Culture and Self.* Cambridge: Cambridge University Press.

———. 1996. "Imaginal Performance and Memory in Ritual Healing." In *The Performance of Healing,* edited by Carol Laderman and Marina Roseman, 91–113. London: Routledge.

Danforth, Loring M. 1989. *Firewalking and Religious Healing.* Princeton: Princeton University Press.

Das, Veena. 1994. "Moral Orientations to Suffering: Legitimation, Power, and Healing." In *Health and Social Change in International Perspective,* edited by Lincoln C. Chen, Arthur Kleinman, and Norma C. Ware, 139–67. Cambridge, MA: Harvard University Press.

Das, Veena, Arthur Kleinman, Margaret Lock, Mamphela Ramphele, and Pamela Reynolds, eds. 2001. *Remaking a World: Violence, Social Suffering, and Recovery.* Berkeley: University of California Press.

Davis-Floyd, Robbie, and Gloria St. John. 1998. *From Doctor to Healer: The Transformative Journey.* New Brunswick: Rutgers University Press.

de Certeau, Michel. 1984. *The Practice of Everyday Life.* Translated by Steven Rendall. Berkeley: University of California Press.

Derrida, Jacques. 1985. "Racism's Last Word." In *Race, Writing, and Difference,* edited by Henry Louis Gates Jr., 329–38. Chicago: University of Chicago Press.

Desjarlais, Robert. 1997. *Shelter Blues: Sanity and Selfhood among the Homeless.* Philadelphia: University of Pennsylvania Press.

Dilthey, Wilhelm. 1989. *Selected Works.* Vol. 1. Edited by Rudolf A. Makreel and Frithjof Rodi. Princeton: Princeton University Press.

Diouf, Mamadou. 2000. "The Senegalese Murid Trade Diaspora and the Making of a Vernacular Cosmopolitanism." Translated by Steven Rendall. *Public Culture* 12:679–02.

Doescher, M., B. Saver, P. Franks, and K. Fiscella. 2000. "Racial and Ethnic Disparities in Perceptions of Physician Style and Trust." *Archives of Family Medicine* 9 (10): 1156–63.

Dray, William H. 1993. *The Philosophy of History.* 2nd ed. Englewood Cliffs, NJ: Prentice Hall.

Dreier, Ole. 2008. *Psychotherapy in Everyday Life.* New York: Cambridge University Press.

Dressler, William. 1993. "Health in the African American Community: Accounting for Health Disparities." *Medical Anthropology Quarterly* 7 (4): 325–45.

Du Bois, W. E. B. 1913. *The Crisis,* July.

Eaton, David. 2008. "Ambivalent Inquiry: Dilemmas of AIDS in the Republic of Congo." In *Postcolonial Disorders,* edited by Mary-Jo DelVecchio Good, Sandra Teresa Hyde, Sarah Pinto, and Byron J. Good, 238–59. Berkeley: University of California Press.

Erlmann, Veit. 1996. "The Aesthetics of the Global Imagination: Reflections on World Music in the 1990s." *Public Culture* 8:467–87.

Families USA. 2002. "Health Coverage in African American Communities: What's the Problem and What Can We Do about It?" December. www.familiesusa.org/assets/pdfs/AfrAmA9acc.pdf.

Fanon, Frantz. 1963. *The Wretched of the Earth.* New York: Grove Press.

Farmer, Paul. 1999. *Infections and Inequalities: The Modern Plagues.* Berkeley: University of California Press.

Fischer, Michael M. J. 2007. "Epilogue: To Live with What Would Otherwise Be Unendurable: Return(s) to Subjectivities." In *Subjectivity: Ethnographic Investigations,* edited by João Biehl, Byron Good, and Arthur Kleinman, 423–46. Berkeley: University of California Press.

Fletcher, M. A. 1998. "L.A., a Sense of Future Conflicts." *Washington Post,* April 7, A1.

Forster, E. M. 1927. *Aspects of the Novel.* New York: Harcourt Brace Jovanovich.

Foucault, Michel. 1965. *Madness and Civilization: A History of Insanity in the Age of Reason.* Translated by Richard Howard. New York: Random House.

———. 1973. *The Birth of the Clinic: An Archaeology of Medical Perception.* Translated by A. M. Sheridan Smith. New York: Vintage Books.

———. 1979. *Discipline and Punish: The Birth of the Prison.* Translated by Alan Sheridan. New York: Vintage Books.

———. 1990. *The Use of Pleasure.* Vol. 2 of *The History of Sexuality.* Translated by Robert Hurley. New York: Vintage Books.

———. 1995. *Discipline and Punish: The Birth of the Prison.* 2nd ed. Translated by Alan Sheridan. New York: Vintage Books.

Frank, Arthur W. 1995. *The Wounded Storyteller: Body, Illness, and Ethics.* Chicago: University of Chicago Press.

———. 2004. *The Renewal of Generosity: Illness, Medicine, and How to Live.* Chicago: University of Chicago Press.

———. 2010. *Letting Stories Breathe: A Socio-Narratology.* Chicago: University of Chicago Press.

Frank, Gelya. 2000. *Venus on Wheels: Two Decades of Dialogue on Disability, Biography, and Being Female in America.* Berkeley: University of California Press.

Franklin, Sarah. 1997. *Embodied Progress: A Cultural Account of Assisted Conception.* London: Routledge.

———. 2005. "Stem Cells R Us: Emergent Life Forms and the Global Biological." In *Global Assemblages: Technology, Politics and Ethics as Anthropological Problems,* edited by Aihwa Ong and Stephen J. Collier, 59–78. New York: Blackwell.

Gadamer, Hans Georg. 1975. *Truth and Method.* London: Continuum International Publishing Group.

———. 2004. "A Debate with Hans Georg Gadamer." In *A Ricoeur Reader: Reflection and Imagination,* edited by Mario J. Valdés, 216–41. Toronto: University of Toronto Press.

Garro, Linda C. 2000. "Cultural Knowledge as Resource in Illness Narratives: Remembering through Accounts of Illness." In *Narrative and the Cultural Construction of Illness and Healing,* edited by Cheryl Mattingly and Linda C. Garro, 70–87. Berkeley: University of California Press.

———. 2003. "Narrating Troubling Experiences." *Transcultural Psychiatry* 40 (1): 5–43.

Garro, Linda C., and Cheryl Mattingly. 2000. "Narrative as Construct and Construction." In *Narrative and the Cultural Construction of Illness and Healing,* edited by Cheryl Mattingly and Linda C. Garro, 1–49. Berkeley: University of California Press.

Gates, Henry Louis, Jr., and Cornel West. 1996. *The Future of the Race.* New York: Knopf.

Geertz, Clifford. 1973. *The Interpretation of Cultures.* New York: Basic Books.

———. 1980. "Blurred Genres: The Refiguration of Social Thought." *American Scholar* 80:165–79.

Giddens, Anthony. 1979. *Central Problems in Social Theory: Action, Structure, and Contradiction in Social Analysis.* Berkeley: University of California Press.

———. 1991. *Modernity and Self-Identity: Self and Society in the Late Modern Age.* Stanford: Stanford University Press.

Ginsburg, Faye D., Lila Abu-Lughod, and Brian Larkin, eds. 2002. *Media Worlds: Anthropology on New Terrain.* Berkeley: University of California Press.

Goldberg, David Theo. 1997. *Racial Subjects: Writing on Race in America.* New York: Routledge.

Good, Byron J. 1994. *Medicine, Rationality, and Experience: An Anthropological Perspective.* New York: Cambridge University Press.

Good, Byron J., and Mary-Jo DelVecchio Good. 1993. "'Learning Medicine': The Constructing of Medical Knowledge at Harvard Medical School." In *Knowledge, Power and Practice: The Anthropology of Medicine and Every-*

day Life, edited by Shirley Lindenbaum and Margaret Lock, 81–107. Berkeley: University of California Press.

Good, Byron, Mary-Jo DelVecchio Good, Sandra Teresa Hyde, and Sarah Pinto. 2008. "Postcolonial Disorders: Reflections on Subjectivity in the Contemporary World." In *Postcolonial Disorders*, edited by Mary-Jo DelVecchio Good, Sandra Teresa Hyde, Sarah Pinto, and Byron J. Good, 1–42. Berkeley: University of California Press.

Good, Mary-Jo DelVecchio. 1995. *American Medicine: The Quest for Competence*. Berkeley: University of California Press.

———. 2007. "The Medical Imaginary and the Biotechnical Embrace: Subjective Experiences of Clinical Scientists and Patients." In *Subjectivity: Ethnographic Investigations*, edited by João Biehl, Byron Good, and Arthur Kleinman, 362–80. Berkeley: University of California Press.

Good, Mary-Jo DelVecchio, Byron J. Good, T. Munakato, Y. Kobayashi, and C. Mattingly. 1994. "Oncology and Narrative Time." *Social Science and Medicine* 38:855–62.

Good, Mary-Jo DelVecchio, Byron J. Good, C. Schaffer, and S. E. Lind. 1990. "American Oncology and the Discourse on Hope." *Culture, Medicine and Psychiatry* 14:59–79.

Good, Mary-Jo DelVecchio, Cara James, Byron J. Good, and Anne E. Becker. 2002. "The Culture of Medicine and Racial, Ethnic, and Class Disparities in Healthcare." In Unequal Treatment: Confronting Racial and Ethnic Disparities in Health Care, edited by Brian D. Smedley, Adrienne Y. Stith, and Alan R. Nelson, 594–625. Washington, DC: National Academy Press.

Gordon, Deborah. 1988. "Tenacious Assumptions in Western Medicine." In *Biomedicine Examined*, edited by Margaret Lock and Deborah Gordon, 11–56. Dordrecht, Netherlands: Kluwer Academic Publishers.

———. 1990. "Embodying Illness, Embodying Cancer." *Culture, Medicine, and Psychiatry* 14:275–97.

Gordon, Deborah, and Eugenio Paci. 1997. "Disclosure Practices and Cultural Narratives: Understanding Concealment and Silence around Cancer in Tuscany, Italy." *Social Science and Medicine* 44 (10): 1433–52.

Gron, Lone, Cheryl Mattingly, and Lotte Meinert. 2008. "Kronisk hjemmearbejde: Sociale hab, dilemmaer og konflikter I hjemmearbejdnarrativer i Uganda, danmark og USA" [Chronic Homework: Social Hopes, Dilemmas and Conflicts in Homework Narratives in Uganda, Denmark and the USA]. *Tidsskrift for forskning I sygdom og samfund*, no. 9: 71–96.

Gupta, Akhil, and James Ferguson. 1997a. *Culture, Power, Place: Explorations in Critical Anthropology*. Durham: Duke University Press.

———, eds. 1997b. "Discipline and Practice: The Field as Site, Method, and Location in Anthropology." In *Anthropological Locations: Boundaries and Grounds of a Field Science*, edited by Akhil Gupta and James Ferguson, 1–46. Berkeley: University of California Press.

Hahn, Robert A. 1985. "Between Two Worlds: Physicians as Patients." *Medical Anthropology Quarterly* 16 (4): 87–98.

Hahn, Robert A., and Atwood D. Gaines. 1985. "Among the Physicians: Encounter, Exchange and Transformation." In *Physicians of Western*

Medicine: Anthropological Approaches to Theory and Practice, edited by Robert A. Hahn and Atwood D. Gaines, .Boston: D. Reidel.

Haller, J. 1970. "The Physician versus the Negro." *Bulletin of the History of Medicine* 44:154–67.

Hallowell, A. Irving. 1955. *Culture and Experience.* Philadelphia: University of Pennsylvania Press.

Hammonds, E.M. 1994. "Your Silence Will Not Protect You: Nurse Eunice Rivers and the Tuskegee Syphilis Study." In *The Black Women's Health Book: Speaking for Ourselves,* 2nd ed., edited by Evelyn C. White, 323–31. Seattle: Seal Press.

Hannan, Edward L., Michelle van Ryn, Jane Burke, Danice Stone, Dinesh Kumar, Djavad Arani, Walter Pierce, et al. 1999. "Access to Coronary Artery Bypass Surgery by Race/Ethnicity and Gender among Patients Who Are Appropriate for Surgery." *Social Science and Medicine* 50:813–28.

Haraway, Donna. 1997. *Modest Witness @ Second Millennium. Female Man Meets OncoMouse: Feminism and Techoscience.* New York: Routledge.

Hebdige, Dick. 1988. *Hiding in the Light: On Images and Things.* London: Routledge.

Hedegaard, Mariane, and Marilyn Fleer. 2008. *Studying Children: A Cultural-Historical Approach.* Berkshire: Open University Press.

Heidegger, Martin. 1962. *Being and Time.* Translated by John Macquarrie and Edward Robinson. New York: Harper and Row.

Herbert, Bob. 2009. "More Than Charisma." *New York Times,* January 24, A1.

Hollan, Douglas. 2001. "Developments in Person-Centered Ethnography." In *The Psychology of Cultural Experience,* edited by Carmella C. Moore and Holly F. Mathews, 48–67. New York: Cambridge University Press.

Holland, Dorothy, William Lachiocotte Jr., Debra Skinner, and Carole Cain. 1998. *Identity and Agency in Cultural Worlds.* Cambridge, MA: Harvard University Press.

Hooks, Bell. 1992. *Daughters of the Dust: The Making of an African American Woman's Film.* New York: New Press.

Hughes-Freeland, Felicia. 1998. Introduction to *Ritual, Performance, Media,* edited by Felicia Hughes-Freeland, 1–28. London: Routledge.

Hunt, L.M. 2004. "Should 'Acculturation' Be a Variable in Health Research? A Critical Review of Research on U.S. Hispanics." *Social Science and Medicine* 59:973–86.

———. 2005. "Health Research: What's Culture Got to Do with It?" *Lancet* 366 (9486): 617–18.

Hunter, Kathryn Montgomery. 1991. *Doctor's Stories: The Narrative Structure of Medical Knowledge.* Princeton: Princeton University Press.

Hurwitz, Brian, Trisha Greehalgh, and Vieda Skultans, eds. 2004. *Narrative Research in Health and Illness.* Malden, MA: Blackwell.

Hyde, Sandra Teresa. 2008. "Everyday AIDS Practices: Contestations of Borders and Infectious Diseases in Southwest China." In *Postcolonial Disorders,* edited by Mary-Jo DelVecchio Good, Sandra Teresa Hyde, Sarah Pinto, and Byron J. Good, 189–217. Berkeley: University of California Press.

Hýden, Lars-Christer, and Jens Brockmeier, eds. 2008. *Health, Illness and Culture*. New York: Routledge.

Ingstad, Benedicte, and Susan Reynolds Whyte, eds. 1995. *Disability and Culture*. Berkeley: University of California Press.

———, eds. 2007. *Disability in Local and Global Worlds*. Berkeley: University of California Press.

Jackson, Michael. 1989. *Paths toward a Clearing: Radical Dmpiricism and Ethnographic Inquiry*. Bloomington: Indiana University Press.

———. 1995. *At Home in the World*. Durham: Duke University Press.

———. 1996. Introduction to *Things As They Are: New Directions in Phenomenological Anthropology*, 1–50. Bloomington: Indiana University Press.

———. 2002. *The Politics of Storytelling: Violence, Transgression, and Intersubjectivity*. Copenhagen: Museum Tusculanum Press, University of Copenhagen.

———. 2005. *Existential Anthropology: Events, Exigencies and Effects*. Methodology and History in Anthropology 11. New York: Berghahn Books.

Jay, Martin. 2005. *Songs of Experience: Modern American and European Variations on a Universal Theme*. Berkeley: University of California Press.

Johnson, Barbara. 1985. "Thresholds of Difference: Structures of Address in Zora Neale Hurston." In *Race, Writing, and Difference*, edited by Henry Louis Gates Jr., 278–89. Chicago: University of Chicago Press.

Johnson, R., S. Saha, J. J. Arbelaez, M. C. Beach, and L. A. Cooper. 2004. Racial and Ethnic Differences in Patient Perceptions of Bias and Cultural Competence in Health Care. *Journal of General Internal Medicine* 19 (2): 101–10.

Kaiser Commission onMedicaid and the Uninsured. 2000. "Health Insurance Coverage and Access to Care among African Americans." Key Facts. June. www.healthpolicy.ucla.edu/pubs/files/HealthInsuranceCoverageandAccess toCareAmongAfrican%20Americans.pdf.

Kapferer, Bruce. 1983. *A Celebration of Demons: Exorcism and the Aesthetics of Healing in Sri Lanka*. Bloomington: Indiana University Press.

———. 1986. "Performance and the Structuring of Meaning and Experience." In *The Anthropology of Experience*, edited by Victor W. Turner and Edward M. Bruner, 188–203. Urbana: University of Illinois Press.

Kleinman, Arthur. 1989. *The Illness Narratives: Suffering, Healing, and the Human Condition*. New York: Basic Books.

———. 2006. *What Really Matters: Living a Moral Life Amidst Uncertainty and Danger*. Oxford: Oxford University Press.

Kleinman, Arthur, Veena Das, and Margaret Lock. 1997. Introduction to *Social Suffering: Essays*, ix–xxvii. Berkeley: University of California Press.

Kleinman, Arthur, and Joan Kleinman. 1991. "Suffering and Its Professional Transformation. Toward an Ethnography of Interpersonal Experience." *Culture, Medicine and Psychiatry* 15 (3): 275–301.

Kondo, Dorinne K. 1990. *Crafting Selves: Power, Gender, and Discourses of Identity in a Japanese Workplace*. Chicago: University of Chicago Press.

Laderman, Carol. 1996. "The Poetics of Healing in Malay Shamanistic Performances." In *The Performance of Healing*, edited by Carol Laderman and Marina Roseman, 115–42. New York: Routledge.

Laderman, Carol, and Marina Roseman, eds. 1996. *The Performance of Healing*. New York: Routledge.

Lakes, Kimberly, Steven R. López, and Linda C. Garro. 2006. "Cultural Competence and Psychotherapy: Applying Anthropologically Informed Conceptions of Culture." *Psychotherapy* 43:380–96.

Lave, Jean. 1988. *Cognition in Practice: Mind, Mathematics and Culture in Everyday Life*. New York: Cambridge University Press.

Lave, Jean, and Etienne Wenger. 1991. *Situated Learning: Legitimate Peripheral Participation*. New York: Cambridge University Press.

LaVeist, T. A., K. Nickerson, and J. V. Bowie. 2000. "Attitudes about Racism, Medical Mistrust, and Satisfaction with Care among African-American and White Cardiac Patients. *Medical Care Research and Review* 57, Suppl. no. 1: 146–61.

Lawlor, Mary C. 2003. "The Significance of Being Occupied: The Social Construction of Childhood Occupations." *American Journal of Occupational Therapy* 57 (4): 424–34.

———. 2004. "Mothering Work: Negotiating Healthcare, Illness and Disability, and Development." In *Mothering Occupations: Challenge, Agency, and Participation*, edited by Susan A. Esdaile and Judith A. Olson, 306–23. Philadelphia,: F. A. Davis.

Lawlor, Mary C., and Cheryl Mattingly. 2009. "Understanding Family Perspectives on Illness and Disability Experience." In *Willard and Spackman's Occupational Therapy*, 11th ed., edited by Elizabeth B. Crepeau, Ellen S. Cohn, and Barbara A. Boyt Schell, 33–44. Philadelphia: Lippincott Williams and Wilkins.

Lawton, Julia. 2000. *The Dying Process: Patients' Experiences of Palliative Care*. New York: Routledge.

Lillie-Blanton, M., M. Brodie, D. Rowland, D. Altman, and M. McIntosh. 2000. "Race, Ethnicity, and the Health Care System: Public Perceptions and Experiences." *Medical Care Research and Review* 57, Suppl. no. 1: 218–344.

Linger, D. T. 1994. "Has Culture Theory Lost Its Mind?" *Ethos* 22 (3): 284–315.

Lock, Margaret. 1996. "Death in Technological Time: Locating the End of Meaningful Life." *Medical Anthropology Quarterly*, n.s., 10 (4): 575–600.

———. 1997. "Displacing Suffering: The Reconstruction of Death in North American and Japan." In *Social Suffering: Essays*, edited by Arthur Kleinman, Veena Das, and Margaret Lock, 207–44. Berkeley: University of California Press.

Lock, Margaret., and Deborah Gordon. 1988. "Relationships between Society, Culture, and Biomedicine: An Introduction to the Essays." In *Biomedicine Examined*, ed. Margaret Lock and Deborah Gordon, 11–56. New York: Springer.

Luhrmann, T. R. 2000. *Of Two Minds: The Growing Disorder in American Psychiatry*. New York: Knopf.

Luria, A.R. 1987. *The Man with a Shattered World: The History of a Brain Wound.* Translated by Lynn Solotaroff. Cambridge, MA: Harvard University Press.

MacIntyre, Alasdair. 1981. *After Virtue: A Study in Moral Theory.* Notre Dame: University of Notre Dame Press.

Mahon, Maureen E. 2000. "Visible Evidence of Cultural Producers." *Annual Review of Anthropology* 29:467–92.

Martin, Emily. 1994. *Flexible Bodies: Tracking Immunity in American Culture from the Days of Polio to the Days of AIDS.* Boston: Beacon Press.

Mattingly, Cheryl. 1994. "The Concept of Therapeutic Emplotment." *Social Science and Medicine* 38 (6): 811–22.

———. 1998a. *Healing Dramas and Clinical Plots: The Narrative Construction of Experience.* Cambridge: Cambridge University Press.

———. 1998b. "In Search of the Good: Narrative Reasoning in Clinical Practice." *Medical Anthropology Quarterly* 12 (3): 273–97.

———. 2000. "Emergent Narratives." In *Narrative and the Cultural Construction of Illness Healing,* edited by Cheryl Mattingly and Linda Garro, 181–211. Berkeley: University of California Press.

———. 2003. "Becoming Buzz Lightyear and Other Clinical Tales: Indigenizing Disney in a World of Disability." *Folk: Journal of the Danish Ethnographic Society* 45:9–32.

———. 2004. "Performance Narratives in Clinical Practice." In *Narrative Research in Health and Illness,* edited by Brian Hurwitz, Trisha Greenhalgh, and Vieda Skultans, 73–94. London: Blackwell.

———. 2006a. "Pocahontas Goes to the Clinic: Popular Culture as Lingua Franca in a Cultural Borderland." *American Anthropologist* 108 (3): 494–501.

———. 2006b. "Reading Medicine: Mind, Body, and Meditation in One Interpretive Community." *New Literary History* 37 (3): 563–81.

———. 2007. "Acted Narratives: From Storytelling to Emergent Dramas." In *Handbook of Narrative Inquiry: Mapping a Methodology,* edited by D. Jean Clandinin, 405–25. Thousand Oaks, CA: Sage Publications.

———. 2008a. "Reading Minds and Telling Tales in a Cultural Borderland." *Ethos* 36 (1): 136–54.

———. 2008b. "Stories That Are Ready to Break." In *Health, Illness, and Culture: Broken Narratives,* edited by Lars-Christer Hyden and Jens Brockmeier, 79–98. New York: Routledge.

Mattingly, Cheryl, and Maureen Hayes Fleming. 1994. *Clinical Reasoning: Forms of Inquiry in a Therapeutic Practice.* Philadelphia: F.A. Davis.

Mattingly, Cheryl, and Mary C. Lawlor. 1998. "Illness Experience from a Family Perspective." In *Willard and Spackman's Occupational Therapy,* 9th ed., edited by Maureen. Neistadt and Elizabeth B. Crepeau, 43–53. Philadelphia: J.B. Lippincott.

———. 2001. "The Fragility of Healing." *Ethos* 29 (1): 30–57.

———. 2003. "Disability Experience from a Family Perspective." In *Willard and Spackman's Occupational Therapy,* 10th ed., edited by Elizabeth B.

Crepeau, Ellen S. Cohn, and Barbara A. Boyt Schell, 69–79. Philadelphia: J.B. Lippincott.

———. n.d. "Re-Situating Cultural Competence." Unpublished manuscript.

Mbembe, Achille. 1992. "The Banality of Power and the Aesthetics of Vulgarity in the Postcolony." *Public Culture* 4:1–30.

Mechanic, David. 2008. *The Truth about Health Care: Why Reform Is Not Working in America.* New Brunswick: Rutgers University Press.

Meinert, Lotte. 2009. *Hopes in Friction: Schooling, Health, and Everyday Life in Uganda.* Charlotte, NC: Information Age Publishing.

Metcalf, Peter. 2001. "Global 'Disjuncture'and the 'Sites' of Anthropology." *Cultural Anthropology* 16 (2): 165–82.

Mishler, Elliot G. 1986. *Research Interviewing: Context and Narrative.* Cambridge, MA: Harvard University Press.

Miyazaki, Hirokazu. 2004. *The Method of Hope: Anthropology, Philosophy, and Fijian Knowledge.* Stanford: Stanford University Press.

———. 2008. "Barack Obama's Campaign of Hope: Unifying the General and the Personal." *Anthropology News* 49 (8): 4–5.

Morris, David B. 1998. *Illness and Culture in the Postmodern Age.* Berkeley: University of California Press.

Mullan, Fitzhugh. 1985. "Seasons of Survival: Reflections of a Physician with Cancer." *New England Journal of Medicine* 313 (4): 270–73.

Obama, Barack. 2004. "2004 Democratic National Convention Keynote Address." American Rhetoric Online Speech Bank, www.americanrhetoric.com/speeches/convention2004/barackobama2004dnc.htm.

———. 2006. *The Audacity of Hope.* New York: Crown.

Ochs, Elinor, and Lisa Capps. 2001. *Living Narrative: Creating Lives in Everyday Storytelling.* Cambridge, MA: Harvard University Press.

Olafson, Frederick A. 1979. *The Dialectic of Action: A Philosophical Interpretation of History and the Humanities.* Chicago: University of Chicago Press.

Olwig, Karen F., and Kirsten Hastrup. 1997. *Siting Culture: The Shifting Anthropological Object.* London: Routledge.

Ortner, Sherry B. 1999. Introduction to *The Fate of Culture: Geertz and Beyond,* edited by Sherry B. Ortner, 1–13. Berkeley: University of California Press.

———. 2006. *Anthropology and Social Theory: Culture, Power, and the Acting Subject.* Durham: Duke University Press.

Paerregaard, Karsten. 1997. *Linking Separate Worlds: Urban Migrants and Rural Lives in Peru.* New York: Berg.

Park, Melissa. 2008. "Making Scenes: Imaginative Practices of a Child with Autism in a Therapy Session." *Medical Anthropology Quarterly* 22 (3): 234–56.

Pepper, Curtis Bill. 1984. *We the Victors: Inspiring Stories of People Who Conquered Cancer and How They Did It.* New York: Doubleday Books.

Petersen, Alan. 2003. "Governmentality, Critical Scholarship, and the Medical Humanities." *Journal of Medical Humanities* 24 (3/4): 187–200.

Polanyi, Michael. 1974. *Personal Knowledge: Towards a Post-Critical Philosophy.* Chicago: University of Chicago Press.

Pollock, Sheldon, Homi K. Bhabha, Carol A. Breckenridge, and Dipesh Chakrabarty. 2000. "Cosmopolitanisms." *Public Culture* 12:577–89.

Porter, Cornelia. 1994. "Stirring the Pot of Differences: Racism and Health." *Medical Anthropology Quarterly* 8 (1): 102–6.

Powell, Jason L., and Simon Biggs. 2004. "Ageing, Technologies of Self and Bio-Medicine: A Foucauldian Excursion." *International Journal of Sociology and Social Policy* 24 (6): 17–29.

Powell, Michael. 2008. "Embracing His Moment, Obama Preaches Hope in New Hampshire." *New York Times,* January 5.

Price, Monroe Edwin. 1999. "Satellite Broadcasting as Trade Routes in the Sky." *Public Culture* 11:69–85.

Rabbani, Juleon. 2008. "Addressing Inequities to Health Care in a Globalized Metropolis: Los Angeles and African Americans." In *Opportunities in Global Health,* edited by Gurinder Shahi and Mana Pirnia, 160–73. Sun Valley, CA: GBI Books; Los Angeles: Global Health Review.

Rapp, Rayna, and Ginsburg, Faye. 2001. "Enabling Disability: Rewriting Kinship, Reimagining Citizenship." *Public Culture* 13 (3): 533–56.

Reverby, Susan M., ed. 2000. *Tuskegee's Truths: Rethinking the Tuskegee Syphilis Study.* Chapel Hill: University of North Carolina Press.

Reynolds, Pamela. 1989. *Childhood in Crossroads: Cognition and Society in South Africa.* Grand Rapids, MI: William B. Eerdmans).

Rhodes, Lorna A. 1995. *Emptying Beds: The Work of an Emergency Psychiatric Unit.* Berkeley: University of California Press.

Ricoeur, Paul. 1984. *Time and Narrative.* Vol. 1. Translated by Kathleen McLaughlin and David Pellauer. Chicago: University of Chicago Press.

——. 1985. *Time and Narrative.* Vol. 2. Translated by Kathleen McLaughlin and David Pellauer. Chicago: University of Chicago Press.

——. 1988. *Time and Narrative.* Vol. 3. Translated by Kathleen Blamey and David Pellauer. Chicago: University of Chicago Press.

Riessman, Catherine Kohler. 2008. *Narrative Methods for the Human Sciences.* Thousand Oaks, CA: Sage Publications.

Rosaldo, Renato. 1989. *Culture and Truth: The Remaking of Social Analysis.* Boston: Beacon Press.

Rose, Nikolas. 2007. *The Politics of Life Itself: Biomedicine, Power, and Subjectivity in the Twenty-first Century.* Princeton: Princeton University Press.

Sacks, Oliver. 1984. *A Leg to Stand On.* New York: Summit Books.

——. 1987. *The Man Who Mistook His Wife for a Hat and Other Clinical Tales.* New York: Perennial Library.

——. 1995. *An Anthropologist on Mars: Seven Paradoxical Tales.* New York: Knopf.

Sahlins, Marshall. 2000. *Culture in Practice: Selected Essays.* New York: Zone Books.

Sargent, Carolyn, and Grace Bascope. 1996. "Ways of Knowing about Birth in Three Cultures." *Medical Anthropology Quarterly* 10 (2): 213–36.

Schafer, Roy. 1981. *Narrative Actions in Psychoanalysis.* Worcester: Clark University Press.

———. 1992. *Retelling a Life: Narration and Dialogue in Psychoanalysis.* New York: Basic Books.

Schechner, Richard. 1990. "Magnitudes of Performance." In *By Means of Performance: Intercultural Studies of Theatre and Ritual,* edited by Richard Schechner and Willa Appel 19–49. Cambridge: Cambridge University Press.

Schein, Louisa. 2002. "Mapping Hmong Media in Diasporic Space." In *Media Worlds: Anthropology on New Terrain,* edited by Faye Ginsburg, Lila Abu-Lughod, and Brian Larkin, 229–44. Berkeley: University of California Press.

Scheper-Hughes, Nancy. 1993. *Death without Weeping: The Violence of Everyday Life in Brazil.* Berkeley: University of California Press.

Schieffelin, E. 1996. "On Failure and Performance: Throwing the Medium out of the Science." In *The Performance of Healing,* edited by Carol Laderman and Marina Roseman, 59–90. New York: Routledge.

———. 1998. "Problematizing Performance." In *Ritual, Performance, Media,* edited by Felicia Hughes-Freeland, 194–207. London: Routledge.

Schleiermacher, Friedrich. 1998. *Schleiermacher: Hermeneutics and Criticism.* Edited and translated by Andrew Bowie. Cambridge: Cambridge University Press.

Scott, James C. 1985. *Weapons of the Weak: Everyday Forms of Peasant Resistance.* New Haven: Yale University Press.

Segal, S. P., R. J. Bola, and M. A. Watson. 1996. "Race, Quality of Care, and Antipsychotic Prescribing Practices in Psychiatric Emergency Services." *Psychiatric Services* 47(3): 282–86.

Sides, Josh. 2004. *L.A. City Limits: African American Los Angeles from the Great Depression to the Present.* Berkeley: University of California Press.

Siegel, Bernie S. 1993. *How to Be an Exceptional Patient: Living with Love and Hope.* New York: HarperAudio.

Smedley, Audrey. 1999. *Race in North America: Origin and Evolution of a Worldview.* Boulder, CO: Westview Press.

Sontag, Susan. 1978. *Illness as Metaphor.* New York: Picador.

Spence, Donald P. 1982. *Narrative Truth and Historical Truth: Meaning and Interpretation in Psychoanalysis.* New York: W. W. Norton.

Spitulnik, Debra. 1993. "Anthropology of Mass Media." *Annual Review of Anthropology* 22:293–315.

Stoller, Paul. 1989. *The Taste of Ethnographic Things: The Senses of Anthropology.* Philadelphia: University of Pennsylvania Press.

———. 1996. "Sounds and Things: Pulsations of Power in Songhay." In *The Performance of Healing,* edited by Carol Laderman and Marina Roseman, 165–84. London: Routledge.

———. 1997. *Sensuous Scholarship.* Philadelphia: University of Pennsylvania Press.

———. 2004. *Stranger in the Village of the Sick: A Memoir of Cancer, Sorcery, and Healing.* Boston: Beacon Press.

Stone, John. 2002. "Race and Health Care Disparities: Overcoming Vulnerability." *Theoretical Medicine* 23:499–518.

Tambiah, Stanley J. 1985. *Culture, Thought, and Social Action: An Anthropological Perspective.* Cambridge: Cambridge University Press.

Tapper, Melbourne. 1999. *In the Blood: Sickle Cell Anemia and the Politics of Race*. Philadelphia: University of Pennsylvania Press.

Taussig, Michael T. 1980. "Reification and the Consciousness of the Patient." *Social Science and Medicine* 14:3–13.

Taylor, Charles. 1989. *Sources of the Self: The Making of the Modern Identity*. Cambridge, MA: Harvard University Press.

———. 2007. *A Secular Age*. Cambridge, MA: Harvard University Press.

Thompson, John B. 1984. *Critical Hermeneutics: A Study in the Thought of Paul Ricoeur and Jürgen Habermas*. Cambridge: Cambridge University Press.

Throop, C. Jason. 2003. "Articulating Experience." *Anthropological Theory* 3 (1): 2–26.

———. 2010. *Suffering and Sentiment: Exploring the Vicissitudes of Experience and Pain in Yap*. Berkeley: University of California Press.

Todd, K.H., C. Deaton, A.P. D'Adamo, and L. Goe. 2000. "Ethnicity and Analgesic Practice." *Annals of Emergency Medicine* 35:11–16.

Traube, Elizabeth G. 1996. "'The Popular' in American Culture." *Annual Review of Anthropology* 25:127–51.

Tsing, Anna Lowenhaupt. 2005. *Friction: An Ethnography of Global Connections*. Princeton: Princeton University Press.

Turner, Edith L.B. 1992. *Experiencing Ritual: A New Interpretation of African Healing*. Philadelphia: University of Pennsylvania Press.

Turner, Victor W. 1969. *The Ritual Process: Structure and Anti-structure*. Chicago: Aldine.

———. 1986a. *The Anthropology of Performance*. New York: PAJ Publications.

———. 1986b. "Dewey, Dilthey, and Drama: An Essay in the Anthropology of Experience." In *The Anthropology of Experience*, edited by Victor W. Turner and Edward M. Bruner, 33–44. Urbana: University of Illinois Press.

Turner, Victor W., and Edward M. Bruner, eds. 1986. *The Anthropology of Experience*. Chicago: University of Illinois Press.

van Ryn, Michelle, and J. Burke. 2000. 'The Effect of Patient Race and Socio-Economic Status on Physicians' Perceptions of Patients." *Social Science and Medicine* 50:813–28.

van Ryn, Michelle, and S.S. Fu. 2003. "Paved with Good Intentions: Do Public Health and Human Service Providers Contribute to Racial/Ethnic Disparities in Health?" *American Journal of Public Health* 93 (2): 248–55.

Waitzkin, Howard, and Holly Magana. 1997. "The Black Box in Somatization: Unexplained Symptoms, Culture, and Narratives of Trauma." *Social Science and Medicine* 45 (6): 811–25.

Weiss, Meira. 1997. "Signifying the Pandemics: Metaphors of AIDS, Cancer, and Heart Disease." *Medical Anthropology Quarterly* 11 (4): 456–76.

Wenner, Jan. 2008. "A New Hope." *Rolling Stone,* March 20.

Wertsch, James V. 2002. *Voices of Collective Remembering*. New York: Cambridge University Press.

West, Cornel. 1993. *Race Matters*. Boston: Beacon Press.

———. 2008. *Hope on a Tightrope: Words and Wisdom*. Carlsbad, CA: Smiley Books.

White, Hayden. 1980. "The Value of Narrativity in the Representation of Reality." In *On Narrative*, edited by W. J. Thomas Mitchell, 117–36. Chicago: University of Chicago Press.

———. 1987. *The Content of Form: Narrative Discourse and Historical Representation*. Baltimore: Johns Hopkins University Press.

———. 1999. *Figural Realism: Studies in the Mimesis Effect*. Baltimore: John Hopkins University Press.

Whitehead, Tony L. 1997. "Urban Low-Income African American Men, HIV/AIDS, and Gender Identity." *Medical Anthropology Quarterly* 11 (4): 411–17.

Williams, Raymond. 1989. *The Resources of Hope: Culture, Democracy, Socialism*. London: Verso.

Wilson, William J. 2009. *More Than Just Race: Being Black and Poor in the Inner City*. New York: W. W. Norton.

Young, Allan. 1995. *The Harmony of Illusions: Inventing Posttraumatic Stress Disorder*. Princeton: Princeton Unversity Press.

Index

Abu-Lughod, Lila, 10, 235–36n4
actions, narrative's role in understanding, 48–50, 239n11
activity theory, 237n1
African Americans: black churches' role for, 24; clinical care in Los Angeles for, 83–84; communication barriers with health care professionals, 28; medicine and construction of black identity, 91–96; race's role in health disparities for, 27–29, 84–87; settlement in Los Angeles, 78–84; slavery's role in defining the black body, 10; socioeconomic class of, 28–29, 86, 89–90, 230; on the Tuskegee syphilis study, 93; uninsured, 87–90
Andrena (case study), 232–33; Belinda as Pocahontas, 176; circulation of her story, 109–12; clinical encounters as border trouble, 98–114, 244n7; the doctor's disappearance, 202–6; emergency-room conflict as a turning point for, 100–102; first meeting with, 1–3, 100; the Halloween party, 167–71; and the healing drama of an encounter with the oncologist, 147–57; hearing of Belinda's diagnosis, 51, 102; hearing of Belinda's impending death, 203; home problems attributed to, 111; medical records vs. Andrena's narrative, 102–5, 108–9; military language in Belinda's

treatment, 63; mind reading by, 150; misreadings in her clinical encounters, 50–51; nightmare of, 3–4; pediatric oncological care navigated by, 12–13; practice of hope after Belinda's death, 220; a therapy session, 157–67; transformative journey of, 155–57; "Yes I Can/No You Can't" game with Belinda, 148, 151–57, 168–71, 204–5
anthropology: biomedicine critiqued by, 240–41n18; culture- vs. experience-centered, 40–41; Geertz on, x; goals of, 9; healing rituals investigated by, 144; linguistic, 30–31; vs. philosophy, x
anticipatory imagination, 15
Appadurai, Arjun, 180–81, 198
Aristotle, 3, 37, 104, 107, 121
autism, 22

Barthes, Roland, 43
Bastide, Roger, 3
Bauman, Zygmunt, 8–9
behaviorism, 42
Belinda (case study). *See* Andrena
Bentham, Jeremy, 56
Bhabha, Homi, 10–11, 13
biotechnologies/biomedicine: anthropological critiques of, 240–41n18; heroic, 66, 241n21; hope produced by, 5; as instrumental, 206; medical imaginary in, 55, 240n17; and modernity, 55–56;

TEXT
10/13 Sabon

DISPLAY
Sabon

COMPOSITOR
Toppan Best-set Premedia Limited

INDEXER
Carol Roberts

PRINTER AND BINDER
Maple-Vail Book Manufacturing Group